D0058690

WAR DOCTOR

WAR DOCTOR

SURGERY ON THE FRONT LINE

DAVID NOTT

INTRODUCTION BY
HENRY MARSH

ABRAMS PRESS, NEW YORK

First published 2019 by Picador, an imprint of Pan Macmillan.

Library of Congress Control Number: 2019944027

ISBN: 978-1-4197-4424-2
eISBN: 978-1-68335-906-7

Printed and bound in the United States

10 9 8 7 6 5 4 3 2 1

ABRAMS The Art of Books
195 Broadway, New York, NY 10007
abramsbooks.com

To Elly, Molly, and Elizabeth with love.

CONTENTS

PREFACE

I have traveled the world in search of trouble. It is a kind of addiction, a pull I find hard to resist. It stems partly from the desire to use my knowledge as a surgeon to help people who are experiencing the worst that humanity can throw at them, and partly from the thrill of just being in those terrible places, of living in a liminal zone where most people have neither been nor want to go.

Since time immemorial man has waged war, usually on his neighbor. As warfare became professionalized, the risk of being injured or killed on the battlefield was borne mostly by soldiers. Wars were fought as a succession of pitched battles, usually away from where people lived, and only the actual combatants were in the line of fire. During the Second World War, however, this began to change, and has continued to do so until today, when the majority of casualties are innocent civilians.

As the size of the group of potential victims has grown, so has the means of wounding or killing them become ever more effective. Thankfully, destruction on the scale of the two atomic assaults visited on Japan over seventy years ago, when hundreds of thousands were killed with a single devastating weapon, has never been repeated. But instead we have multiple and increasingly powerful delivery systems for rockets, missiles, bombs, and bullets, all of which are designed to inflict terrible damage on the human body. And wars most affect those who are worst equipped to deal with them: people who are poor or disenfranchised, living in inadequate or unsanitary conditions with few of the amenities we take for granted in the West. War can make an already difficult existence impossible.

There are doctors and nurses, good doctors and nurses, all over the world—the desire to make medical care your life's work seems, thank goodness, to be a pretty consistent ambition for a percentage of every population. But extreme events, whether a war or a natural disaster, stretch the boundaries of performance and what is possible. Injuries are more devastating; the windows of opportunity to intervene become shorter; resources are scarcer or run out sooner; medical personnel are more stressed, and are often in danger themselves. Even the best-trained surgeons in peacetime will be shocked by what they see in a war zone, as I was myself; it takes time to build up the skills and experience necessary to cope with the many different challenges a trauma surgeon will face.

For reasons I will try to explore in this book, I have for over two decades now spent much of my time volunteering to go to dangerous places to help those who have been affected by events that are, very often, utterly beyond their control. I have ventured into other people's wars many times—in Afghanistan, Sierra Leone, Liberia, Chad, the Ivory Coast, the Democratic Republic of the Congo, Sudan, Iraq, Pakistan, Libya, Gaza, and Syria to mention a few. Sometimes my work has been carried out in well-provisioned hospitals away from the fighting and sometimes in poorly equipped field hospitals on the front line—what we call "austere environments," where there are few investigatory tools such as X-ray machines or CT scanners to rely on.

Why do I keep going back to areas of pure misery and heartache? The answer is simple: to help people who, like you and I, have a right to proper care at this most precarious time of their lives.

What do we do when a little child traps her finger in a door and cries, and we are the only one there? We scoop that precious little person up into our arms. We feel the pain, we offer reassurance that everything will be OK, and we show love and tenderness; the act of cuddling transmits a feeling of protection. It says, "I'm here now and I'm going to look after you, and make you better."

That same human response is exactly what is required when you face a patient with terrible injuries in a conflict zone. That patient wants comfort and protection from what has happened. The initial doctor-patient relationship must provide that and instill a feeling of confidence that the doctor will be able to help, do the right thing, and take away the pain of injury.

Hospitals can be emotional places at the best of times, and in war environments all sensitivity is heightened. It is vital to adopt and radiate an air of confidence and strength. I am much better at that now than I used to be. However, the stakes are high because there are often weapons around, tensions are raised, and the rule of the gun overrides the rule of law. I have been in many dangerous situations and there is no doubt I am lucky to have stayed alive.

The Geneva Conventions are there to provide protection both for all those injured *and* to all those who provide treatment in war. In 2016, I organized a demonstration in London against the indiscriminate bombing of hospitals in Syria and in the world's other war zones. Hospitals must be protected and respected. To bomb and destroy hospitals is not just sinful, it is evil—evil because it is claimed by the perpetrators to be justifiable and intentional. In Syria there were over 450 attacks on hospitals in the first six years of the conflict there, nine out of ten of them perpetrated by the Syrian and Russian governments. In some months of the conflict there have been attacks on medical facilities practically every day. Not only is performing these acts evil—so is denying that they are happening.

Organizing a public demonstration, or being interviewed on television to campaign for humanitarian corridors, or setting up a foundation to spread specialist expertise about trauma surgery—these would have been impossible things for me to contemplate when I was a young consultant in the early 1990s. They are the acts of a man my younger self would not have recognized—except it is still me, and we are both the product of my Welsh upbringing and all the myriad factors that shape a personality.

The campaigning and the teaching that drive me now are a function of all my experiences, but in particular my experiences in recent years in Syria. I have made three major trips there since 2012, along with other visits to the border zone, and in that period my life has changed profoundly. I began seriously to collate and share the knowledge I had acquired over my career to help other doctors, especially doctors from countries at war. I began to get seriously angry about the inability of the major powers to prevent hospitals and medical staff from being targeted in environments where they were simply trying to save lives. And, most miraculously of all,

I became seriously involved with the woman who I knew I wanted to spend the rest of my life with, married her, and became a father.

I have been to other places since 2012, but Syria is the thread that runs through this most extraordinary period of my life, the seam to which I keep returning. These trips have been the most extraordinarily fulfilling, frustrating, and dangerous of all.

INTRODUCTION

Is the practice of medicine a business or is it a vocation? Where does the balance lie between doing well and doing good? The hypocrisy of doctors—money and medicine are rarely far apart—has long been the stuff of satire and criticism. The dictionary definition of the word "vocation" talks of a "special urge" or of a "calling"—but there are many reasons why people choose to become doctors, and most of them have little to do with altruism. Doctors, of course, will all differ as to where they find a balance between money and morality, just as they will vary as to where they find a balance between compassion and scientific detachment, another tightrope they have to negotiate.

As patients, we like to think that our doctors are dedicated professionals, entirely devoted to us. Our anxiety—for who is not anxious when they go to see a doctor?—has us invest them with supernatural powers and the highest moral standards, as a way of reducing our fear. It is inevitable that we are often disappointed—doctors are only human, and life is still a fatal condition.

But despite this, the idea of the doctor as hero is deeply ingrained, and many doctors—especially in the early years of their careers—like to think of themselves as heroic. They usually soon discover that medical heroism is mainly a matter of hard work and long hours—inevitable parts of medical practice—even though in countries such as America and England there is now talk of the need for unheroic "work-life balance" and the dangers of "physician burnout." But what are we to think of doctors who put not just their well-being, but their very lives at risk, by working in conflict zones? Are they thrill-seeking narcissists or true heroes?

David Nott is one such doctor. The list of countries where he has worked as a trauma surgeon is a catalog of all the most deadly and dangerous places in which a doctor could work over the last thirty years—Bosnia, Afghanistan, the Congo, Rwanda, Iraq, Gaza, and, most recently and most terribly, Syria.

As readers will discover in *War Doctor*, he is in many ways a modern-day saint—equivalent, at least to outside observers, to the martyred men and women of the early Church, who gave their lives for something greater than themselves. But this book is written from the inside, with honesty and considerable insight.

Nott describes his wish to work in war zones as "a kind of addiction." He has come very close indeed to being killed on several occasions. After the first such occasion, in Sarajevo, he writes, "I felt elated, exhilarated, euphoric. I had never felt more alive; it was as if I had been reborn." The risk of death, and the cruelty he has often had to witness—such as watching women being stoned to death in Afghanistan under the rule of the Taliban—can bring ecstatic reward (of a sort) as well as horror. At least as a doctor, perhaps he is less vulnerable to the guilt that many war correspondents—a breed of adventurers with whom Nott admits he has much in common—experience when they have to impotently watch such scenes.

The idea of altruism as being in pure opposition to selfishness is nonsense. A cynic—which I am not—might say that the extreme altruism displayed by people like Nott is really a form of narcissism. In reality, of course, altruism and egotism are two sides of the same coin and reflect our intensely social natures as human beings. We need other people, and we need to be needed. We can find intense fulfillment in putting the lives of others ahead of our own (as we do with our own children), and most of us long for a cause, even if it is only to try to stave off ecological disaster by feeding the few remaining sparrows in our backyard. Doctors like Nott, who lead such extreme lives, are a glorious expression of this deep human need, although you may well wonder what drives them.

The paradox of extreme altruism—that it is simultaneously selfish—finds a parallel in the fact that most surgeons take up surgery because they find it exciting. Most doctors do not want to become surgeons and indeed often regard them as a necessary evil. Where the surgeon is excited, other doctors would simply be frightened. Many doctors recoil from shedding blood, even if in a good cause, and find it hard to suppress their natural empathy—empathy, in distinction from sympathy, meaning our ability actually to feel for ourselves other people's feelings. You could not operate on patients if you yourself actually felt what they were feeling. Surgeons, obviously, do not suffer from this problem—though I do not know whether this is from lack of empathy or because the excitement of operating enables them to switch off their empathy when necessary (and in some cases permanently). The dividing line between fear and excitement, of course, is hard to define—in terms of neurophysiology, the same parts of the brain are active in both states. The difference lies in whether you feel in control or not, and surgeons, it seems to me—a surgeon myself—find an intense pleasure in feeling that they are in control. (Sometimes I suspect that this reflects a deep insecurity and fear of being out of control.) But what makes the surgery exciting is your fear that the operation might go horribly wrong—so the surgeon's selfish search for excitement in fact has an altruistic result.

This awkward balancing act, between thrill-seeking and compassion, is very apparent with expatriate doctors working in war zones, especially with regard to their local colleagues, who cannot fly away back to the comforts of the modern world when they feel like it, having had their hit of excitement and doing good. Nott is well aware of this, and it is perhaps one of the factors that drove him, as a sort of expiation, into the dangers of working in Syria, where he was in constant danger of being captured (and probably beheaded) by ISIS. He tells us that he spent much of his time there in a state of abject terror.

Nott quotes a saying from the Koran (also to be found in the Talmud) that he who saves a life, saves the world. This is not a philosophy to which the admirable organization Médecins sans Frontières (MSF) and other aid organizations can easily subscribe—we live in a world of limited resources and must make hard choices as to which lives can be usefully saved and which are better abandoned. Nott falls out with MSF as he makes desperate (and yet successful) efforts to save the lives of two children deemed beyond help. I am far too much of a coward to have risked my life by working in war zones, but I have worked in many impoverished countries, such as Nepal and Sudan. I learned early on that with the limited resources available to me, I could not help every child with a brain tumor that I saw. I can remember several occasions when, despite the parents' desperate pleading, unlike the Good Samaritan, I did not cross the street. It hurt—and even now, years later, the memory still does.

A surgeon's life, especially for somebody like Nott, comes at a price. What is so touching about his book is that what eventually trips him up in his dance with Death—risking his own life to save others (and sometimes failing)—is that in his fifties he falls deeply in love. As he tells us, this—combined with the loss of the feeling of invulnerability that he had when young—provokes a complete breakdown. His altruism for his patients is now in conflict with his own, more immediate desires. But love (surely one of the most misrepresented and often selfish of human emotions) prevails, and he becomes a father. He inevitably has to reorganize his priorities, and yet continue to help his colleagues in Syria. Which he does, with great success. At one point this involves dinner with the Queen of England—a moving and yet hilarious scene that I will leave readers to discover for themselves.

Just what the inner demons were that so drove him, and perhaps still drive him (you rather hope they no longer do), he does not say. Perhaps he himself does not know. But the world is a much, much better place to have people like David Nott in it.

Henry Marsh
October 2019

– 1 –
THE BOMB FACTORY

The London 2012 Summer Olympics were in full flow, with Team Great Britain winning a record number of medals and the country basking in the reflected glory of our athletes and a successful Games. It was hard to imagine that only a few hours' flight away an entire country was descending into violent anarchy.

I was busy with my day job for the National Health Service. For most of the year I work at three hospitals in London: St. Mary's, where I am a consultant vascular (blood vessels and circulation, from the Latin *vas*, for vessel) and trauma surgeon; the Royal Marsden, where I help the cancer surgeons from various specialties such as general surgery, urology, facio-maxillary, and gynecology remove large tumors *en bloc*, which then require extensive vascular reconstruction; and the Chelsea and Westminster, where I am a consultant laparoscopic (keyhole) and general surgeon. But alongside this work, in most years since the early 1990s I've also done a few weeks' trauma surgery in a war zone. I monitor the news avidly, keeping an eye out for developing hotspots, knowing at some point soon an aid agency is likely to ask me to help.

When I get such a call, my heart begins to race and I develop an irrepressible urge to remove any obstacle that might prevent me from going. My immediate response is always, "Give me a couple of hours and I will come back to you." The call might come while I'm operating or assisting a colleague, or I might be holding a routine outpatient clinic. Wherever I am and whatever I am doing, the desire to go is always intense and almost overwhelming. But I can't say yes every time. I might get a couple of requests a month from different agencies, and could easily be a full-time volunteer, but I have to earn a living, too. I do receive £300 or so for a month's fieldwork, but mostly that's spent on everyday expenses.

Before agreeing to anything, I call the surgical manager at Chelsea and Westminster, where my contract is held, and explain that there's a humanitarian crisis in which I've been asked to help. I then request immediate unpaid leave for the time I'll be away. There is usually no objection, "as long as you can sort out your clinics and your operating and your on-calls." Indeed, I have never yet been turned down. No doubt the carrot of taking unpaid leave while maintaining all my commitments helps to allay any anxieties the NHS might have!

So I didn't need asking twice when, during the summer of 2012, a call came from the head office of Médecins Sans Frontières (MSF) in Paris, asking if I would be prepared to work in a hospital they'd set up in Syria. I made the usual arrangements at home, packed my things, and got on a plane to Turkey.

Like most people, I knew Syria was a country in the Middle East that had steered clear of the conflicts that had beset many of its neighbors—three of the countries it borders are Iraq, Lebanon, and Israel, hardly oases of calm. For most of my lifetime Syria had been a closed, slightly secretive sort of place, but peaceful, where more adventurous Western tourists sometimes went on holiday, with a population known for its warm and hospitable nature.

It's a truism I'll return to that many of the countries I've volunteered in have collapsed into chaos after a challenge to authoritarian rule. Nature might abhor a vacuum, but warmongers love them. In Syria's case the authoritarianism was provided by the Assad family, who had ruled over the country since taking power in a bloodless coup in 1970. The current president, Bashar al-Assad, had taken over after the death of his father, Hafez, in 2000—winning 99.7 percent of the vote that confirmed his assumption of power. The Assad family are leading lights in the minority Alawite sect, a branch of Shia Islam in a country where nearly three-quarters of the population are Sunnis. There was something of a cult of personality around them, with pictures of Hafez and Bashar the decor of choice in many offices and stores. Their grip on power was, in time-honored fashion, reinforced by a notoriously brutal secret police, conspicuous in their ubiquitous sunglasses and leather jackets.

My acquaintance with Syria went back a long way: my father had had a Syrian trainee called Dr. Bourak in the 1970s, whom my dad said was the best resident he had ever worked with, and I had also met a young Dr. Bashar al-Assad while he was an ophthalmic resident at the Western Eye Hospital in London in the early 1990s. We were discussing a patient who had eye problems from a small clot that had come off the carotid artery. He seemed very pleasant and respectful—little did I know that our paths would cross again many years later.

In Syria the plates had begun to shift in 2010, the year demonstrators in Tunisia took to the streets to complain about a host of grievances including high levels of corruption, unemployment, and lack of freedom of expression. Early in the new year Tunisia's long-serving president was deposed, and others across North Africa and the Middle East, experiencing similarly bad government, began to take notice. There were sustained protests in Morocco, Algeria, and Sudan throughout early 2011, and then across to Iraq, Lebanon, Jordan, and Kuwait. And in five other countries—Libya, Egypt, Yemen, Bahrain, and Syria—the phenomenon that became known as the Arab Spring led to serious insurgencies, the toppling of regimes, or full-blown civil war. So far, only Tunisia has managed to turn the turmoil into positive democratic change: many of the other countries are arguably much worse off than before.

In Syria, suppression of the protests calling for President Assad's removal was particularly brutal. In my opinion the whole civil war could have been avoided, or quickly curtailed, if the regime had responded to the protests in a more moderate way. In March 2011 some children sprayed anti-government graffiti on walls in the southern city of Daraa; Assad's response was to have his security forces detain the children and torture them. Thousands of protesters took to the streets in response. On March 22, Assad's forces stormed the hospital in Daraa and occupied the building, positioning snipers on the roof. As the protests escalated, the snipers began their work. A surgeon named Ali al-Mahameed was killed as he tried to attend to the wounded, and when thousands of mourners turned up at his funeral later that day, they too were shot at. Snipers would remain stationed on the roof for another two years, firing on sick and injured people who were simply trying to get treatment.

As protests erupted all over Syria, the country's medical system became a lightning rod for the divisions tearing Syrian society apart. Those opposing the regime—mostly Sunnis, from among whom the Free Syrian Army emerged—found that seeking treatment for injuries sustained in the fighting became almost as dangerous as the fighting itself.

The healthcare system was weaponized by the regime. Government-run hospitals functioned as an extension of the security apparatus: it was reported that staff still loyal to Assad would routinely deal with minor injuries by carrying out amputations as a form of punishment. Protesters who had been wounded and were awaiting treatment were often taken from the wards and spirited away to be tortured and killed.

In the first year of the uprising a documented fifty-six medical workers were either targeted by government snipers or tortured to death in detention facilities. In July 2012, Assad passed a new law against failing to report anti-government activity, in effect making the medical treatment of anyone not actively supporting Assad a criminal offense. This was the kind of pressure medical staff across the country were having to face simply to do their job.

I flew to Istanbul and then on to Hatay, the airport near to Reyhanlı, the closest Turkish town to the Syrian border. I was then taken to the MSF safe house in Reyhanlı and given a briefing on the mission, the latest security alerts and escape routes in case of emergency evacuation. The following day I was picked up by a Syrian driver and a local Syrian logistician and taken to a checkpoint just before the border where I was given a false name and signed in as such and was given some papers. The driver then took me to the border, which was under the watchful eye of the Turkish military, who also checked my papers. We crossed the border, which at that time was just a barbed-wire fence, and waited for the Syrian car to take me to the MSF hospital in Atmeh. We passed the fledgling refugee camp, which had a few thousand people in ragged tents with poor sanitary conditions. Although the tents were disheveled, I was surprised to see the people inside were very well-dressed with clean shoes, and must have taken pride in their appearance. I am sure that they did not realize that their refugee status was just the beginning of a miserable existence that they were to endure for years to come. Médecins Sans Frontières (known as Doctors Without Borders in the US), a medical humanitarian organization with which I had worked on several occasions, had taken over a large walled villa in the town and converted it into a hospital, code-named Alpha, as it was the first such facility they set up in Syria. The house was large and well-proportioned and belonged to a man who happened to be a surgeon himself who was working in Aleppo. The rooms had been repurposed in anticipation of growing demand: the dining room became our operating room, the living room was our emergency room, where patients were first assessed, and the kitchen housed the sterilization unit. The first and second floors became our wards, with about twenty beds, and the staff accommodation was on the top floor—although when I arrived it was so warm we used to sleep on the roof, under mosquito nets. A mix of Syrians and foreign volunteers like me, we'd lie up there, exhausted after a nonstop shift, watching the jets streaking overhead and staring up at the stars in the inky night sky.

I quickly settled into a rhythm and began to feel useful. We'd get up early, have a meeting with the project manager, who would brief us on the security situation that day, where the latest fighting was concentrated, and so on, and then we'd do our ward rounds. I was very pleased to see that Pete Matthew, an excellent doctor I'd worked with before, was there, too. A consultant neurosurgeon from Dundee, Scotland, Pete had some years earlier been very keen to try his hand at humanitarian work. Back in 2002, with my colleagues Pauline Dodds and Jenny Hayward-Karlsson, I had run a training course sponsored by the British Red Cross to train British surgeons to work in war zones and Pete had been one of the delegates. We became great friends and had stayed in touch ever since.

After the ward round in Atmeh we'd have breakfast and then start on any scheduled operations: to begin with, in this early stage of the war, we were not overrun with casualties and there was still time to do elective or follow-up surgery for people whose lives were no longer in immediate danger.

But things soon heated up, and before long there was a great deal of significant emergency surgery going on—we began to see lots of gunshot wounds and fragmentation injuries as the regime began shelling civilian homes and firing rockets from helicopters. People were facing not only the primary risk of a direct hit, perhaps killing them outright or resulting in a catastrophic amputation, but also the secondary risk of fragmentation or shrapnel injuries as the metal shell casings flew in all directions and bits of buildings hit by a missile became deadly projectiles.

Every now and then, at any time of day or night, we might hear the blaring of a car or pickup truck's horn in the distance, getting louder and louder as the vehicle sped toward us with its cargo of victims. The horns acted as a siren, and we'd know to get the emergency room ready so we could assess the patients and decide who needed to go straight into surgery. On one occasion, the first patient to need our help turned out to be the wife of a local bomb-maker. At that time there were a lot of small factories opening up in Atmeh that were making explosives. These were fairly crude devices and few of the people making them knew what they were doing—they were mostly working at home, making it up as they went along, and putting their own families at terrible risk.

The woman's husband had apparently been making a bomb in their kitchen when it had detonated prematurely. The whole house was destroyed, the bomb-maker killed, and his wife rushed to us with a fragment injury to her lower left leg. She was hemorrhaging significantly from the wound, which required a tourniquet to be placed immediately on the thigh.

The anesthesiologist took a quick blood sample and put it through our very basic hemoglobinometer, a device which measures the red cell count in blood. It confirmed that she had a hemoglobin of 4 grams per liter (the normal amount of hemoglobin—the stuff that carries oxygen in the blood—is between 12 and 15g/L). It was clear she had lost a great deal of blood. He quickly established her blood group and then went to get a pint of fresh blood of the right type from our dwindling supplies. Then, on the other arm, he set up a saline drip to replace some of the fluid that she had lost.

All this happened on the operating table in the dining room. The nurse in charge set up the gurney with sterile drapes and instruments as the patient was given general anesthesia. It was impossible to assess the wound properly as there was arterial bleeding, most likely from the superficial femoral artery in the leg. There was a large dressing on the top, which was acting as a local compression. I scrubbed up and prepared to operate.

One of the Syrian assistants, who didn't speak much English, was helping to lift the leg. As I prepped the limb with iodine, I asked the helper to take off the pressure dressing. The bleeding by this time had stopped, and there was a large clot overlying the wound. With the patient now draped and prepped, I started the procedure by making an incision below the tourniquet, high on the leg, so that I could get a clamp on the artery before exploring the wound. After gaining proximal control of the blood vessel I then went down to have a proper look. I tentatively put my finger into a large hole just above her knee joint and felt an object in there which I assumed was a piece of metal—a fragment from the bomb, or maybe a bit of her house.

In this kind of scenario it is always important to go very carefully, putting your finger into the wound slowly and cautiously because there may be fractured bone, which can be as sharp as shards of glass—the last thing you want is a needlestick injury without knowing the blood status of the patient. In this environment there was perhaps less concern about HIV or hepatitis, but it is a common mistake not to assume the worst.

Probing gently with my finger, it didn't appear to be the usual jagged piece of metal or fragment but a smooth, cylindrical object. Very carefully I grabbed it with my fingers and pulled it out. I held it up to examine it, and the Syrian helper who was with me took one look and went pale. He obviously knew what I was holding and blurted out, "*Mufajir!*" before turning tail and leaving the room.

The anesthesiologist and I looked at each other. Was I holding some sort of bomb? In that instant, I froze as I wondered what on earth I should do next. It became extremely quiet—all I could hear was the soft hiss of the ventilator pumping oxygen into the patient's lungs. The anesthesiologist shuffled away, moving across to the corner of the room behind one of the cabinets. By now my hands were shaking, I was in danger of dropping whatever it was, and I realized I had to do something. I decided to take a deep breath and walk out of the operating room as carefully and slowly as I could. I needed the anesthesiologist to open the door for me and jerked my head in its direction to show him what I wanted, hardly daring to speak. He said to wait, as he was sure somebody was going to come very shortly—thankfully he was right, and as I deliberated for a few more seconds the door opened and in came the Syrian helper with a bucket of water. He put the bucket on the floor next to me and he and the anesthesiologist ran to the safety of the next room. With my heart pounding, I carefully put the object into the bottom of the bucket, feeling the cold water seeping into the sleeve of my green scrubs, and very gingerly took it outside.

Mufajir means "detonator." It was hard to tell if it was live or not. I was told later that it probably would not have killed me, but it would most likely have blown off my hand—not the end of my life, maybe, but certainly the end of my career, and at the time the two were much the same thing.

It wasn't the last time I had a run-in with homespun explosives. Most of the fragmentation wounds from bombs that we were receiving were from the effects of amateur bomb-makers. Several times throughout the mission, we would receive young girls and boys at the hospital who had lost one or both of their hands. Some had severe facial injuries as well, and, even more pitifully, some had dreadful eye damage that rendered them blind. Many times I would go to the ward and hear the sobbing of parents holding their five- or six-year-old, who would never see them again or touch them with their fingers. It was utterly heartbreaking.

Although all around us there were people coming to terms with being at war, in the house we felt pretty safe. We didn't really take much notice of the building opposite, which seemed to be full of young men in dark combat fatigues, often carrying weapons. I suppose if I thought about it at all, I assumed it was some sort of training facility for the Free Syrian Army. We used to watch them kneeling after the mosque's call to prayer began at around 4:30 in the morning, and knew that they could see us going about our business, too. There was something very romantic about that moment; I would lie awake on the roof, listening to the beautiful voice singing from the mosque. The air at that early hour was sweet with a crisp coldness—

there was a sense of complete tranquility as the sky gradually lightened. By seven o'clock in the morning it was too hot to lie awake on our rubber mattresses, which made it easy for us all to get up and wait our turn for the shared toilet and shower in the building.

The sunsets were equally beautiful. More often than not the evening sky was just a vast swathe of deep blue, with the occasional wispy cloud. The sun cycled through an array of startling colors as it sank down and set between two small mountains on the horizon; it was a wonderful spectacle to watch.

On one such evening, the rest of the team had gone down to the village swimming pool. Feeling self-conscious and a little overweight at the time, I decided not to join them and to go upstairs to the roof for a rest. The sunset was particularly striking, so I decided to take a photograph of it. I'd been doing these missions for many years by this time, and I knew the rule that one should never take photos on a mission with MSF. However, over the years I have always taken clinical photographs and videos for teaching purposes—with the patient's permission, of course—often using a GoPro camera mounted on a headband. And I am very pleased that I did, because without doubt this archive of images has become a major educational tool for the teaching work I do now. And everyone took pictures, all the time—the rule, such as it was, was very widely ignored.

I set up my camera and spent quite a bit of time fiddling with the time-lapse function to get the best shot. As I was doing so I looked down into the street below and noticed someone I recognized—Dr. Isa Rahman, whom I had met at the Turkey-Syria border a few weeks before. I waved to him and he waved back. He had recently qualified from Imperial College and was working with a charity called Hand in Hand for Syria, which had set up a clinic in Atmeh.

I turned back to my camera, which was on the wall overlooking the street and the buildings around us, but focused on the golden horizon far into the distance. After I'd taken a few photos I was startled by the sudden appearance of the hospital's logistician, who burst out onto the roof having run upstairs and told me to stop immediately. He was scared and pale and could hardly speak coherently. I was oblivious to the fact that several floors below me at the entrance to the hospital were about twenty armed men who had suddenly forced their way in. They wanted my camera, thinking I had been taking pictures of them.

"No, no," I protested, "I was just taking pictures of the sunset!"

The aggrieved men were the devout fighters from next door, who had been watching me from a distance. It emerged that they weren't FSA at all but belonged to some jihadi group. The logistician had negotiated with them very quickly that he would get my camera and take it downstairs to show them what was on it. He told me that I must give it to him immediately—they were threatening to overrun the hospital within two minutes if they did not get the camera. I duly gave it to him and sat nervously on a chair with my heart sinking into the pit of my stomach, wondering what would happen next.

The logistician was gone for about fifteen minutes. I stood up and looked over the wall down onto the street below and caught Isa's eye again. I motioned to him to try and see what was going on downstairs, and perhaps do something to help. He nodded to me and walked toward the hospital.

Twenty minutes after beckoning Isa, the logistician reappeared and gave me my camera back, much to my surprise, as I had expected never to see it again. Fortunately there were no images of the jihadis on it, otherwise I would definitely have been taken away for interrogation and God knows what else—but despite the images being entirely innocent, the jihadis had said they wanted to take me anyway. Thankfully, Isa had eventually persuaded them to leave.

I now know that I owe Isa a great deal: shortly after this incident these young fighters abducted another MSF expat, who was held for several months. I never saw Isa again, and was very upset to find out that he was killed about twelve months later, dying from a shell injury sustained while he was working at his clinic in Idlib, which was blamed on the Syrian government forces.

I'd had any number of close shaves by this stage of my career, but this one was memorable more in hindsight—I later realized it was my first encounter with the organization now widely known as Islamic State. It has been given various names, including Daesh, an acronym of the Arabic version, but since my run-ins with its members happened in Syria, I'll refer to it as ISIS (Islamic State of Iraq and Syria).

The photo debacle would come back to haunt me in a different way, too. But at least the pictures were good.

Every so often the mission team would change as one of the doctors or nurses would leave and another would arrive. Sometimes it was a relief for the team that people did move on; no doubt that in a very high-stress environment some people do crack under pressure. You can tell they are not as happy as they were when they arrived; some become a lot quieter, others more vocal. Some even become slightly irrational.

One of the senior nurses who was running the ward was, in my view, beginning to lose sight of the reason we were all there. Pete had done a really difficult operation on a fragmentation injury and was now anxious that there might be a leak from one of his intestinal anastomoses (joins) within the young man's abdomen. In this situation the abdomen becomes extremely painful and its lining, the peritoneum, becomes inflamed. This results in diffuse peritonitis, causing an involuntary spasm of the muscles, which become board-like in nature, like a tabletop. This patient had obvious signs that this had occurred, and Pete and I discussed taking the patient back into surgery. I told the nurse that this was what I was going to do. But she disagreed—she insisted that we needed to take the patient in an ambulance across the border into Turkey for him to have a proper operation there. She started to shout at us in front of other patients and became quite hysterical, demanding that we not operate.

I have no qualms at all about working in a team. From the most junior person up to the most senior, we all have opinions on how best to treat the patient. No one is infallible; it is quite possible to miss a clinical sign or mistake an observation, which will sometimes be brought to light by the most junior person in the room.

When someone actively makes a judgment that is out of their remit, however, then it becomes a problem. Of course, it would have been possible to have called an ambulance to transport the patient to the border, but the journey from Atmeh to the border is slow and protracted, and the pain and distress would have been too great. We discussed the case with Alpha's project manager and in the end took the man back to the operating room and fixed him up.

I wasn't sorry to see the back of that nurse, but usually it is sad to see people go, as with our German emergency physician, who had been excellent. However, I was delighted that his replacement was to be my previous intern at Charing Cross Hospital, Natalie Roberts, who has subsequently become a shining light in humanitarian work and with MSF. As our new emergency physician, she would look after our makeshift emergency room in the living room. It looked out onto a patio, on which there was room for about six beds. Here she would examine patients before surgery, and this was also our overflow area if we had a mass-casualty event and needed more space.

Only a few days after her arrival there was another explosion in a house near the hospital. Again, it was the home of an amateur who was making bombs in cylindrical metal containers about the same size as an old-fashioned bottle of dish soap. At 10:30 in the morning we heard the horns start blaring, getting louder and louder as they approached.

An entire family of eight arrived: mother, father, and six children. They had been praying together in the backyard of their house. As the father prostrated himself, a device had fallen out of his pocket and detonated. All eight family members were brought through the outside door of the hospital onto the patio, where we began to try to make sense of a tangled mess of body parts.

All six of the children were dead, as well as their mother. The father, the bomb-maker, had severe fragmentation injuries to his arms and legs. Some were fairly superficial but others had gone much deeper. We had no X-ray machine available and all the diagnostics had to be made through clinical findings alone—basically, having a good look and making a decision yourself.

Natalie was examining the patient. A small, highly charged fragment with a lot of energy had burst into his chest and caused internal bleeding. This can come from a fractured rib, from an intercostal vessel lying between the ribs, from the lung, or—worst-case scenario—from the heart.

She correctly diagnosed that the man had a significant amount of blood within the chest cavity, which needed removing using a chest drain. This is a tube that is placed through the armpit area via the ribs into the chest cavity—it allows blood and air that is not within the lung to be evacuated, thereby letting the lungs expand and so improve breathing. Natalie seemed to be getting on with this very well, and was also cleverly taking blood out of the chest using a special filter and placing it in another bag to infuse back into the patient.

When anybody comes into an emergency room the first thing we do is called the primary survey—looking at the basic parameters that can save lives, which we in the international community code as CABCDE.

The first "C" stands for catastrophic hemorrhage. If the patient is bleeding significantly then the first thing to do is to try to stop it, either by direct pressure or using a tourniquet, a tight binding with a belt or strap between the heart and the open wound. Sometimes the source of the bleeding isn't obvious, though—it might be coming from somewhere hidden like the chest, the abdomen, or pelvis. If your clinical examination has ruled out the arms and legs as the source, both front and back, then, if the patient is shocked and pale, the bleeding must be coming from somewhere we cannot apply pressure. We then make a decision as to whether or not the patient needs to be taken directly to the operating room.

The next check is "A" for airway, to confirm there is no obstruction to the flow of oxygen to the lungs. Then come the lungs themselves—"B" for breathing, to make sure the lungs can expand properly and provide oxygen to the body. The lungs could be bruised, or be compressed with blood or air, requiring a chest drain.

The second "C" stands for general circulation and a quick assessment of blood pressure by feeling the pulses, while "D" is for disability, the most likely being neurological disability caused by head injuries. "E" stands for exposure—checking the rest of the patient and also understanding the temperature of the environment. To do this, it is important to remove as many of the patient's clothes as possible, so they can be examined front and back.

As I watched Natalie putting in the chest drain, I noticed that, although this man's pants had been partially cut off with a pair of scissors, there was something sticking out of his pocket. It was a cylindrical object, about the size of an aerosol can. Suddenly, it fell out of his pocket onto the floor. It was another bomb.

We all watched as if in slow-motion as the object bounced on the hard, tiled floor of the emergency room and spun in the air on the rebound. Astonishingly, one of the male Syrian interpreters in attendance displayed lightning-quick reactions and did the best David Beckham kick I have ever seen, booting the bomb straight through the open patio door. It didn't explode, presumably because there was no detonator inside, but it was a lesson for us all. We should have checked the patient more thoroughly first—but we had all been so shocked at the carnage wrought on his family that we just got down to work.

War zones are completely different from routine life at home, and it is very easy to become blinkered and not take care of oneself, such is the focus on the patients. But extra precautions must be taken at all times to try to limit the risk of making a mistake. You have to have a different bit of your head switched on—you can't take your normal NHS mind-set to a war. In more well-established hospitals everyone would be checked for weapons with a handheld metal detector before being allowed in—in one of the hospitals where I had worked in northern Pakistan a few months before going to Syria, even the volunteer doctors and nurses were checked when they arrived. But we didn't have one in Atmeh, and had to deal with whoever came in, whoever they were.

I was reminded of a bomb-maker I'd had to work on while I was in Pakistan: a Taliban fighter who'd been injured making improvised explosive devices (IEDs) for use against coalition forces across the border in Afghanistan. He came in and I operated on him, and saved his life. I am often asked how I can square my humanitarian work with saving the life of someone who might go on to make something that kills British soldiers or innocent civilians. It's a valid point, of course, and every war surgeon has to wrestle with the conundrum at some stage. But actually it's quite simple: I don't get to choose who I work on. I can only try to intervene to save the life of the person in front of me who is in desperate need of help. Usually I have no idea who they are or what they have done until afterward anyway—but even if I did know, nothing would change. I rationalize it by thinking, *Well, maybe that Taliban guy or this ISIS fighter will find out his life was saved by a Western, Christian doctor, and that might make him change his outlook.* Some people may consider this naive, but that's how it is.

It wasn't all bomb-makers and the disastrous effects of these amateur explosives that we were dealing with, though. The Syrian regime was increasing its airstrikes on civilians all the time. The dining room/operating room would be in use for about eighteen hours a day as we carried out emergency operations of all kinds on people of all ages. At the same time, we also slowly became a referral center for reconstructive surgery.

One such case was very close to home, as the patient was the man who owned the house that was now Hospital Alpha. As I mentioned, he was a surgeon himself, and had been injured in a missile attack while working in Aleppo. At that time it was possible to drive from Atmeh to Aleppo in about forty-five minutes—when I went back a year later, it took over three hours with all the checkpoints that had been put in place. He was driven fast along the straight road back to his own house. A large fragment of a bomb or building had ripped through his left arm and taken out the bones around his elbow including the arteries and veins. He needed significant reconstruction. Pete and I reestablished the blood supply to his arm with a long segment of vein from his leg and realigned the bones as best we could with an external fixator.

While we were doing this, I became aware of a significant commotion outside, and heard someone demanding in English to be let in. Normally no one was allowed inside the operating room while surgery was in progress, so I let him stew outside as I finished up. Stripping off my gloves, I went out to see what all the fuss was about and found myself face-to-face with a man who claimed to be the vice president of a charity called Syria Relief. He said my patient was a very important person in the Syrian community and that I must release him into his care.

"And who are you?" I said, rather annoyed.

"I am Mounir Hakimi, an orthopedic registrar from Manchester," he said quite grandly.

"Well, I am David Nott, a *consultant* surgeon from London," I shot back.

I refused to let him into the operating room as the patient was still recovering, and as we argued back and forth the testosterone levels rose and things got pretty heated. Luckily an American doctor of Syrian extraction interrupted us and smoothed things over. It was finally agreed that the owner of the house could be moved across the border to Turkey, but only once I was satisfied he was stable enough to travel. He went to Turkey for postoperative care and I was pleased to find out that he recovered well, without requiring any more surgery. It has been a joy to meet him again on my further missions to Syria and I feel a sense of pride every time I see him.

It was not to be my last meeting with Mounir, and as my mission neared its end I could hardly imagine how important he and his native country would become in my life. I knew I would be back. Syria and its people had entered my heart and soul—we had done a lot of good work in a relatively short space of time, saving many lives and also laying the foundation of future care.

In fact this mission epitomized everything I had come to crave in such work—the satisfaction of making a difference; of helping ordinary people; the challenge of self-reliance when working in an austere environment; the camaraderie of dedicated people who share your values—and the odd bit of danger just to spice things up.

The urge to get out there and help still burned strong, and would grow even more intense over the next few years. But where does that urge come from? I suspect it was laid down long ago, and triggered by two formative events experienced by a young man just beginning his career in medicine.

- 2 -
TWO EPIPHANIES

The journey toward danger began somewhere safe. In fact, probably the safest place I've ever known, somewhere I still regard as a kind of haven.

My grandparents' house in Trelech, a small village fifteen miles north-west of Carmarthen in Wales, was where I spent my earliest and happiest childhood years. My grandparents, called Mamgu and Datcu in Welsh, lived in a tiny terraced house at the top of a hill on which the village was built, surrounded by the most beautiful countryside. My mother, Yvonne, had grown up there with her eight siblings, all living on top of each other. It was one of those villages where everyone knew everyone's business. Neither she nor her parents had ever ventured beyond Carmarthen until the day her father drove her all the way to Newport so she could study to become a nurse.

First there was the small business of teaching herself English—only Welsh was spoken at the house in Trelech. But my mother had guts. She was determined to do something with her life and had been inspired in part by meeting the district nurse who had delivered one of her sisters.

Both my parents were what we would now call "healthcare professionals," and the urge to make things better must have run deep—one of my earliest memories is of burning myself on the house's wood-burning stove, aged about two, and of the care and love Mamgu showed as she nursed my injured hand.

I have very vivid memories of my young life in Trelech—helping Datcu in his garage as he worked on machinery from the village, with the strong smell of grease and hundreds of tools and vehicle parts scattered around the floor. He was a bit of a local Mr. Fixit, always tinkering with something, welding, or mending. I remember the air outside being redolent of farmyards, proper rural smells, but also the fresh, clean scent of the countryside, and that I was fascinated by the well fifty yards beyond the garage, which always seemed to produce fresh water. I can still conjure in my mind the outdoor fragrance of my grandfather's clothes—I used to love pressing my nose into the folds of his coat, immersing myself in all it represented.

It was a simple house, defined by simple things, but no less profound for that. Mamgu would chop wood with an ax and the logs would be used on the stove. Apart from Mamgu and Datcu, many of my mother's younger brothers and sisters still lived there, and although it was crowded, I suppose I was spoiled rotten, especially by my young aunts. My main memory from those early years is of fun and laughter and love—and also a deep connection with Wales. I didn't realize it at the time—it was all I knew—but speaking Welsh around the dinner table was another bond, both with one another and with our community. The sense of belonging and being surrounded by family love made us very secure. And the simplicity of the way we lived—not in luxury, by any means, but not hankering after things we couldn't have, or being led astray or feeling we were missing out on anything—was deeply ingrained.

It was a very Welsh childhood, and to me completely magical. It was the mold I came from, by which I have always been indelibly marked. It was the making of me.

It is only since I have become a father myself, quite late in life, that I have come to understand why I lived with Mamgu and Datcu in Trelech, and not with my parents.

My mother had gone to Newport to pursue her dream of becoming a nurse, and it was while she was there that she met my father, Malcolm Nott, a junior doctor. Malcolm was born in the city of Mandalay, right in the middle of what was then Burma, the son of an Indian army officer and a Burmese mother. This was 1955, and of course there were some raised eyebrows at her beginning a relationship with a man from South Asia.

Nott is hardly a typical South Asian name and even now my father's surname makes no sense to me. There have been many stories of how he acquired it. My father's father told me that during the first Afghan war, in 1840, General Sir William Nott led the British forces. He had an Indian batman who took his name. Another story was that my father's great-grandfather was a railway engineer from Hereford who was seconded to help build the Indian railway and stayed in India and married a local woman. I've tried, but haven't been able to substantiate either story.

After Japan's invasion of Burma in 1942, Malcolm led his mother and younger brother across the dangerous mountain border into India (present-day Bangladesh). His elder brother was in the army, and was captured by the Japanese and forced to work on the Burma–Siam railway. He died of malnutrition at the age of twenty-two.

His father, my paternal grandfather, was a communications officer who had been seconded to the British army as a Japanese–English interpreter, working in Singapore among other places before the invasion. His close liaison with the British promised him a better life after the war.

Once in India, my father trained at Madras Medical School, and when he qualified his father told him to go to England to seek his fortune—and also to find him that better place to live that he'd been promised (or promised himself). So my father left home and everything he'd ever known to sail to a new life in Britain, part of that great influx of postwar immigration. He worked for the Post Office in London before landing a job at the Royal Gwent Hospital in Newport. Almost immediately, he met my mother. A few months later they were married and she soon fell pregnant.

Toward the end of her pregnancy my mother went home to Trelech. However, she developed septicemia and was admitted to Priory Street Hospital, Carmarthen, where I was born by Cesarean section in July 1956. We both almost died. My mother didn't want to give up her nursing training, but because she had been absent from the course for longer than she had anticipated, she was told she had to start again from the beginning.

So, with a four-year program to complete and my father still earning very little as a junior doctor, while moving around a lot, often on short-term placements here, there, and everywhere, they decided to let me grow up in the most beautiful place on earth with the most beautiful people on earth—in Trelech with my Mamgu and Datcu, Sam and Annie. And that was where I stayed until I was four years old.

The idyll had to come to an end, though, and when my parents felt settled enough to take me away from Trelech, effectively to begin a new life, it was painful and traumatic for all concerned. Like my mother when she left for Newport, I spoke only Welsh. Trelech was all I'd known. It was my anchor. Although my mother did visit us from Newport, Trelech was home, and Mamgu and Datcu the ones who looked after me. I can remember them both crying, and I'm sure I was wailing for all I was worth, too. I can still picture their sad faces through the back window of our car as we drove away, out of Wales and across the border to England.

We lived for a while in Stoke-on-Trent, and then, when I was about six, moved to the village of Whittington near Worcester. The contrast between this new life and the warmth and laughter of Trelech came as an enormous shock. For the first time in my life I felt alone. I had no siblings, and no prospect of any—it wouldn't have occurred to me to ask if my parents planned to have any more children, and I don't remember any discussion of it. In fact, a relative told me much later that even having me came as a bit of a surprise.

I now spent a lot of time on my own. My father was working around the clock, trying to advance his career, and I didn't see much of him until later, when I was established at primary school. I remember trying to make friends with the boy next door, who was around my age but didn't seem all that interested. One day I decided a charm offensive was required and I went to his house having gathered up all my toys, presenting them to him like some sacrificial offering. My parents soon found out and told me off, making me take them all back.

Since I hadn't seen much of my dad in very early childhood, we were only now getting to know each other. He used to tell me stories of the war, of his brother and father and how his own derring-do had saved his mother from being carried downstream when they were crossing a fast-flowing river during their escape to India. I was transfixed by these stories of faraway lands and I could tell he too yearned for those times and the people he'd left behind.

He also fed my growing passion for model airplanes, often bringing home three or four at a time. These were Airfix kits, each a box full of tiny plastic parts, a tube of glue, and an instruction booklet showing how they all fit together. I used to love making them, painting each component with the stipulated color from my little pots of Humbrol acrylic paint before letting it dry and then bonding it to its neighbor. I suppose it was an early example of the manual dexterity that has served me well as an adult—they were very fiddly, requiring a lot of patience and application.

The models were mostly of Second World War aircraft, and by the age of about eight I had literally hundreds of these planes hanging by cotton threads from the rafters in the ceiling of my bedroom, where Dad would help me pin them up once they were ready. There'd be whole squadrons of Spitfires and Hurricanes, poised to swoop down on a bank of Luftwaffe bombers out on some terrible sortie—my flashlight would become the ground searchlights of London, raking back and forth to identify the enemy as I fought long and complicated mock-battles in my imagination. I even had a favorite pilot I'd invented, an RAF ace called Dirk, who flew a Bristol Beaufighter and could always be relied upon to take out the last Messerschmitt Bf 109.

Looking back, it seems a rather lonely thing to be doing, perhaps even a bit sad. I suppose it was an unusual childhood, but it didn't seem so at the time, and any feelings of loneliness I had would have been half-formed, not fully recognized for what they were. It was just what I knew—along with keeping out of the way of my parents when they argued, which they did a lot. But I could tell the difference between the happiness I'd known in Wales and what I was feeling now, which was quite a long way from happiness, if not its opposite. To my great joy, though, we went back to Wales every summer for the holidays, and sometimes at other times too, and it was always a fantastic tonic to be back there.

I was too young to understand properly the root of my parents' occasional flare-ups, but they were both strong-willed people and I guess had all the anxieties that young parents face. There were frequent fights, and the odd flying dish. And family matters were not straightforward—my mother disliked my paternal grandfather and the feeling was mutual. It can't have been easy either, being an interracial couple in postwar Britain, at a time when attitudes about race, by no means perfect now, were very different.

My grandfather, the Indian army officer, had been very strict with my father, and he certainly inherited some of that disciplinarian streak. He'd return from work and if some misdemeanor or other was reported to him he'd say, "David, it's time to chastise you," and I would get a real beating, his beautiful healing hands turning into weapons as I was clouted. My mother also had a temper. They loved each other, but it seemed to take a long time for them to work out how to *be* with each other.

After Worcester we moved on to Rochdale, just outside Manchester. My father was by this time a consultant orthopedic surgeon. We were now thoroughly middle-class and I went to a grammar school in Oldham.

I did not enjoy school life at all. I had to endure lots of racist comments and received little attention from the teachers. I languished at the back of the class and my academic potential, such as it was, was not nurtured. I did not feel clever and was not made to feel clever. One of my reports even went so far as to say that I would turn out to be a failure. I felt nobody really cared for me. But far from being a bad thing, I have remembered that feeling all my life and it has shaped my personality—I know what it is like to not be wanted and to feel abandoned.

As with my model planes, though, aviation offered another way out. I joined the Combined Cadet Force (CCF) at school, with a particular interest in the Royal Air Force, and walked around with the top button of my shirt undone, swaggering as I imagined a fighter pilot would do.

Indeed my flying career started as a sixteen-year-old RAF cadet being taught to fly a glider in West Malling in Kent by the amazing Second World War fighter-pilot Ray Roberts, who would become my hero after he told me of his daring nighttime sorties in his Lysander, dropping off SOE agents in darkened fields in France. I went on to get my private pilot's license, followed by a commercial pilot's license and eventually an airline transport pilot's license; I flew, believe it or not, a Learjet 45 for Hamlin Jet for around ten years. I still hold a single-engine piston rating, a multi-engine piston rating, an instrument rating, an instructor rating, and a helicopter license, all current.

As a youth, flying became a passion. I was so enamored that I wanted it to be my career. But my father had other ideas, and insisted I should apply for medical school, which in turn dictated my A-level choices of Biology, Physics, and Chemistry. He was very determined that I should become a doctor, sometimes chasing me up the stairs to do my homework or even sitting with me in my room while I studied. I'd even scrubbed up to assist him a couple of times when he was operating on private patients—something that would never be allowed to happen today—and I can't deny I was fascinated by those early experiences. There was a lot riding on it, but I had a backup plan—I had my eye on a Royal Navy helicopter pilot course if things didn't work out.

They didn't. Although I didn't exactly fail my A levels, my grades were awful, and certainly nowhere near good enough to get me a place at university to study medicine. You might think it was a subconscious psychological ploy on my part, underperforming so I could go off and fly helicopters. But I was devastated.

I remember the three of us—Mum, Dad, and me—all in tears as we looked at my grades and considered the consequences. I went out into the yard and tried to make sense of it all. Yes, I could have had more support along the way—but had I given the impression that this was what I really wanted? Had I shown my teachers that I cared, that I wanted to succeed? If people thought I'd been coasting, why should I expect help from them? I was furious with myself. Tramping around our yard, I resolved there and then that I was not going to be made to look a fool ever again.

By the time I came back into the house I knew exactly what I was going to do. I went straight back up to my bedroom and pulled down my A-level Physics textbook. *I'll do it myself*, I thought—and from then on I did work hard, although I didn't do it entirely alone, as a kind teacher called Alex Robinson offered to give me some extra instruction before I re-sat my exams.

Oddly, this crisis also seemed to act as a balm on my parents' relationship—the arguments took a back seat to my progress, and by the time the exams came around I was in a completely different frame of mind, and much better prepared. This time I passed well enough to win a place to study medicine at the University of St. Andrews.

The next three years in Scotland, for what they called the "pre-clinical" part of my medical training, were fantastic. I really blossomed at university, and the difficulties and failures of my teenage years seemed to evaporate.

Suddenly I had lots of friends, including girlfriends for the first time, and a busy social life. St. Andrews is a small place, easy to get around, and there always seemed to be lots going on.

Although I hadn't yet discovered my "vocation" as a surgeon, I was increasingly fascinated by the very wide range of disciplines we were covering. As first-year medical students, we had to learn about the human body, how it works, how it fits together, what makes it run (and what makes it stop running). The technical side of me enjoyed the mechanics of it, and the body is indeed a bit like a machine. If you maintain it properly and give it the right fuel, it will work well. Stop giving it fuel, or the wrong fuel, and let bits of it fall into disrepair, and you'll have problems.

Much of our time was spent in anatomy class, where we'd work on a cadaver while learning about different parts of the body. It sounds odd, looking back on it, but we actually used each cadaver for a whole year—in the first year we began with the head and neck, then in the second year we worked on the torso of another person, and in the final year the arms and legs of someone else. I got to know those three bodies pretty well.

At first it was shocking and strange, of course, to see them—it was the first time many of us had ever seen a dead body. In my very first class I saw a corpse with his arm sticking out at an odd angle, and I felt so disconcerted that I dissolved into fits of giggles. It was shock, of course, but then I felt embarrassed at having been shocked.

All students acclimate to the business of working with and cutting into dead bodies at their own rate. It does take a while to get used to, but it's an essential part of the training. Some people don't ever get used to it, though, and decide to focus on a different aspect of medicine or do something else entirely.

But that was never going to be me. I was aware of the enormous privilege of using someone's actual body to work on and learn from. They had agreed to donate their remains to science and it was the least we could do to show them respect and to try to learn as much from them as we could. We use fresh-frozen cadavers now, bodies that are put on ice almost immediately after death and then defrosted if and when required, but back then they were kept submerged in large vats of formaldehyde. I never saw the room where they were stored in this way—the porters brought them up for us before class—but it must have been a creepy place.

Even now, after being a surgeon for nearly thirty-five years, I still have to steel myself, to an extent, before making that first incision: it is a violent act, after all. But, back then, once the dissection or whatever it was had begun, I found that the body stopped being a "dead person" and became more like a machine for me to explore and examine. There's a procedure I learned later called the "clamshell," where you cut into the thorax and lift it up out of the way, a bit like opening the hood of a car. Once the hood is open, it becomes much easier to engage with the technical challenges of whatever is wrong. I have discovered since that there is a huge difference between cutting someone open in order to make them better and seeing someone whose body is open or damaged because it has been pierced by a bullet or shrapnel.

St. Andrews was a revelation. It was a kind of bubble, but I liked what I found there—the novelty of feeling fulfilled, challenged, my world expanding both intellectually and socially. Once I'd had a taste of these things I didn't want to let them go. I nearly repaid the university by burning it down, though: my great friend and housemate, Johnny Woods, and I had some friends over for a party and a candle set fire to some curtains, the flames then spreading quickly to the whole dorm. The fire department came and put it out, but not before a lot of damage had been done, including to me—I was badly burned. Later, having been dosed up on morphine, I heard someone playing Led Zeppelin's "Stairway to Heaven" through the walls, and thought in my drugged daze that maybe I was on the way there myself.

In 1978 I moved to Manchester for the next three years of my training, on what they called the "clinical" side. Instead of studying anatomy and working with cadavers, this taught us how to find out what was wrong with someone, learning how to examine a patient, taking a history of the symptoms, and arriving at a diagnosis.

I really enjoyed my clinical years. I loved talking to patients, getting to know each of them as a person rather than an illness. But it was not an easy start. A few weeks into clinical work I got to know a female patient on the ward on my first surgical rotation. She was wonderful and I looked forward to seeing her every day and following her through her treatment. She had lung cancer, and required a procedure called a pneumonectomy. We developed such a rapport that I asked the consultant if I could stay with her while she had her operation.

I was as excited as she was when the day arrived. It was the first time I had ever gone into an operating room apart from with my father. I stood in the corner as she was prepared and draped: she was positioned on her side, and I watched with fascination as a huge incision was made in her chest. Every now and then the consultant allowed me to look in, but made a performance about me not touching anything, saying I would be asked to leave if I got in the way.

About two hours into the operation there was an expletive from the surgeon. I watched in horror as blood started to pour from the woman's chest onto the floor. The whole ambience of the OR changed. Suddenly, it felt cold and impersonal. I watched as panic set in and everyone seemed to be shouting. I was told to leave. Not knowing what else to do, I went home.

The following day I discovered that the lady had died on the operating table. It was an enormous shock—I can see her smiling face to this day. It was the first time in my life that someone I knew had died.

This experience had a significant effect on the whole of my first clinical year. I wasn't sure if I was up to the emotional strain of losing a patient I had gotten to know. I began missing lectures and clinical work and ended up failing the end-of-year pathology exam. My heart just wasn't in it. During the microbiology re-sit, rather than discussing bacteria and viruses, the examiner and I talked about why I was having to re-sit the exam. All my anxieties came out in those twenty minutes, and, having answered only a simple question about gas gangrene, I was told, to my amazement, that I had passed. I will never know why the examiner made it so easy for me; perhaps he sensed there were better things to come.

The second year of clinical training was much happier. We spent five nine-week rotations in various specialties, and my favorite was the nine weeks I spent in Hull on obstetrics. We also learned the art of midwifery. I personally delivered twenty-seven babies and performed a number of episiotomies—making a small cut in the lower part of the vagina to avert a more damaging tear during delivery. I found that I was able to sew up the episiotomy with my left hand and as well as my right—it turns out I am ambidextrous, something that has helped me no end in my career as a surgeon.

As a medical student I had always treated qualified doctors with reverence, seeing them as remote and rather austere figures. But on that rotation in Hull I met a wonderful senior house officer called Dr. Caroline Broom. She was such fun to be with, so down-to-earth and natural. She made patients laugh, and it made me realize how a doctor should be. It wasn't just about taking medical histories and examining patients' bodies—it was about connecting with them as people. She taught me a lot about doctoring, not least that practicing medicine well required not just knowledge but empathy and a sense of humor.

At the end of that year, we were allowed to go on an "elective"—a chance to study overseas. I chose to go to Singapore, Malaysia, Thailand, and Burma, mainly because I wanted to see Changi Prison in Singapore, where my grandfather had ended up during the Second World War, and also to visit the Thanbyuzayat War Cemetery in Burma, to lay a wreath given to me by my father for his brother Herbert, who was laid to rest there. It was a wonderful trip, on which I learned a lot—and not only about medicine.

The last year of clinical training was tough, with many hours spent studying late into the night, on top of the clinical work on the wards. But it paid off. I graduated with distinction in medicine and pediatrics in my final exam. So, at the end of my three years in Manchester I had finally qualified and could call myself a doctor. But what kind of doctor did I want to be?

Sometimes a distinction is drawn between those in "medicine" and those in "surgery," to show the difference between doctors who diagnose and prescribe, and those who diagnose and operate. I knew already that the technical aspects of surgery appealed to me more than diagnostic puzzles and I felt that I had inherited a good pair of hands from my orthopedic surgeon father, but was still not completely settled on it—and would have been utterly astonished then to have discovered how much time I would later spend operating.

Once you qualify you begin to climb the greasy pole toward being a consultant, or an attending physician as it's known in the States—and it's worth remembering that everyone in the UK is a "junior doctor" until they become a consultant, which means that some very senior and experienced people are described as "junior." There are roughly three stages before you have a shot at a consultancy—you begin as an intern (called a house officer or junior house officer), then work up to registrar (resident), and, finally, senior registrar (chief resident). When I qualified, the registrar and senior registrar ran the whole emergency surgical on-call. It was almost viewed as a failing on the part of the registrars if they had to call the consultant and junior surgeons performed the majority of all the emergency surgery. Surgery in the 1980s was a trial of sleep deprivation, of how much you could take before you broke. Most of the time we were totally exhausted—on call two nights out of three and working ridiculous hours. In the absence of European Working Time Directives, we would work an average of over 140 hours per week. You could be up all night operating and then have to work all the following day; it was the norm. You were also expected to be able to sit and pass the primary fellowship exam of the Royal College of Surgeons of England, which was considerably tougher than any other exam I had ever sat, before or since. It was not unheard of to find that most of the best surgeons of the day had sat the primary fellowship exam two, three, or four times. I was no different; it took me four attempts before I passed. The goal, however, was to get your next job, keep learning, and move up the ladder.

I still wasn't sure which specialty to choose for my further career until one formative night on call, when I was back in Manchester working as an intern in the neurosurgery unit of the Royal Infirmary. There was no second-year intern and the residents all lived twenty-five miles or so outside the city. One of them, Peter Stanworth, decided it would be a good idea to teach us juniors a procedure that would buy a bit of time if he was at home and had to drive in in his old and very slow car.

Only a few weeks into my time in neurosurgery the interns were taught how to perform burr holes, a technique used to reduce pressure on the brain caused by internal bleeding. Patients who have had a head injury sometimes also have a condition called extradural hematoma—the dura being the lining underneath the cranium that protects the brain. The thinnest part of the skull is above the cheekbone in front of the ear and the middle meningeal artery is just underneath it. If this part of the skull is fractured by a hard blow, the artery bleeds and produces a blood clot, which presses on the dura and compresses the brain. Because the brain is housed in what is in effect a tight box (the cranium), it has nowhere to go except through the only opening in the cranium, which is down the spinal column, into the neck. This opening contains the part of the brain that controls respiration. When it gets squashed, breathing stops and the patient dies. But if you can get to the dura by drilling into the skull, the pressure that's built up inside has an outlet, and the blood that has been pressing on the brain is released. It can be a lifesaving intervention.

Nowadays, there is an electric drill for doing this, but back then (and even still, in the developing world) we used a handheld drill called a Hudson Brace. It has two drill bits; the first is called the perforator and the second bit is the burr. It requires some force to get through the bone, so you need to brace yourself—standing with one leg forward as if about to push a heavy object. The patient's head is usually held steady in a clamp, or sometimes held firmly by a colleague. You go in with the perforator, which makes a V-shaped hole, stopping every now and then to check your progress through the cranium—you don't want to go in too far and hit the brain itself—and wash away any blood with saline. Once the perforator has done its work you follow with the burr drill to make the hole wider and to expose the dura.

In brain trauma there are two types of hemorrhage. Because an extradural hematoma only causes pressure on the brain from outside the dura, if it's relieved quickly then the patient will make a complete recovery, because there is no actual brain injury. The bleed that occurs *under* the dura is called subdural and can be due to actual brain injury and therefore does not have such a good overall prognosis.

On this particular night, I was playing *Space Invaders* in the junior doctors' lounge with some colleagues when I took a referral from Withington Hospital about a lady who had fallen and fractured her skull. Her level of consciousness was reducing significantly and it was felt that she needed to be transferred to the neurosurgical center at the Royal Infirmary, since there was no CT scanner at Withington. I phoned Peter, the registrar, who told me to admit the patient for a scan.

At around 9:00 p.m. the patient arrived but her condition was deteriorating very rapidly. She had started what we call "Cheyne-Stoking," an abnormal pattern of breathing known as Cheyne-Stokes respiration in which the patient adopts a kind of stop-start breathing, with occasional pauses when it looks like they have stopped breathing completely. It indicates that the mid brain is under pressure and being forced down into the spinal column. The on-call anesthesiologists had to very rapidly put a tube down her windpipe to help her breathe.

I pushed her on a gurney down the corridor from the ER to the CT scanner, which I thought showed a massive extradural hematoma. Normally this kind of swelling has a particular shape—extradural hematomas are convex while subdural ones, where the pressure has built underneath the dura, look concave. This one was so big it was hard to tell what shape it was. I phoned Peter again and gave him the news that she was deteriorating in front of my eyes.

"Well," he said, "I've taught you what to do, get on with it."

The hairs on the back of my neck stood up. Having qualified only a few months before and having done a surgical job for only a matter of weeks, I rang the on-call surgical nurse and told her I wanted to open the neurosurgical OR to do an emergency burr hole. She told me that the emergency team were already upstairs with the professor of surgery—he had come in specially to do a renal transplant, and I would have to wait.

I knew that if I waited, my patient would die. So for the first time in my career, I decided to fight for my patient. I wasn't going to be deterred, or bullied by authority.

"I don't care," I said, "I need the emergency team in the operating room immediately." The professor of surgery was the one who would have to wait—he could do his operation after I had finished mine.

Suddenly a Scottish lilt came over the phone.

"Do you know who you're talking to, sonny?" came the reply. "You are lucky I haven't started. I'll send them down and they will be with you soon. A word of advice: stay calm." I couldn't believe it—here I was, the most junior surgeon in the hospital, being given such great encouragement from the most senior. I had no idea how profound those two words were to become, and how they would resonate throughout my life. I can still hear those words echo in my head, especially in times of severe anxiety: "Stay calm."

Within twenty minutes of my call the patient was wheeled into the operating room. Normally we'd be scrubbing up, putting on our masks and gowns, but there was so little time I could only manage to put on some surgical gloves. Because it was so unusual for such a young doctor to perform neurosurgery, word had quickly gotten around the hospital that I was about to operate, and people started wandering in to watch. There must have been about twenty people in there, curious to see how I got on, and having an audience did nothing for my nerves.

With enormous trepidation, and with the hairs on the back of my neck still at attention, I wielded the scalpel. I pushed the knife carefully into the side of the woman's head. I then separated the skin and underlying tissues of the cranium, picked up the perforator and adopted the stance to start drilling, expecting a torrent of blood to come out having hit the clot. But there was no blood. After a while, I picked up the burr drill and proceeded to make the hole bigger, again hoping to hit the jackpot. I could see the dura by now, and it was white—there was no blood there either, and no extradural hematoma.

Oh no, I remember thinking. *What do I do now?*

Then, to make matters even worse, the radiographer leaned over and whispered, "Dave, Dave—other side!"

I'd been drilling on the wrong side of the head.

Battling a sense of impending doom I took a deep breath, quickly went around to the other side of the head and proceeded to do the same operation.

Again, there was no extradural hematoma. However, there was a significant blueness to the dura, indicating that in fact most likely there was a *sub*dural hematoma. This also can occur with a significant head injury and rather than the artery bleeding it is due to significant venous bleeding in the space between the brain and the dura. I could see a kind of blue/red jelly, which suggested this was the darker venous blood rather than the bright-red arterial stuff. I duly cauterized the dura and then made another incision. Finally came the torrent of blood I'd been looking for, all over my pants and shoes.

Within seconds, the patient began to improve: her blood pressure, which had been sky-high, began to fall, and her breathing started to regulate. I was so exhilarated that I performed a further posterior burr hole and washed the entire clot away with saline. As I did this, Peter walked in, saw where I was up to, and, together, we proceeded to finish the operation after he had performed a craniotomy, which involves removing a large part of the cranium to expose the brain and stop the bleeding.

I remember feeling a sense of absolute elation, and revelation, as we finished up. It was the first of two epiphanies at this stage of my career. From that moment on, I knew that I wanted to be a surgeon. I was amazed that a simple act of surgery could pull a patient back from the brink of death.

It was above all a sense of power. First the exercise of power, when I overruled the professor of surgery, making a call on whose case was more important. But that was minor compared with the breathtaking nature of the intervention, the saving power of surgery if you have acquired the necessary techniques to resolve or prevent the effects of a particular physical problem.

This, I thought, *is what it's all about. This is what I want to do with my life.*

It was also an early lesson in the power of decisiveness. As a surgeon you often need to make quick and clear decisions, and sometimes, of course, the stakes could not be higher—it can quite literally be a matter of life and death. But I now knew I had the wherewithal to act decisively, and to back myself and my judgment. This too was enormously empowering.

I was on cloud nine after this experience and got into bed at around one in the morning with a feeling I had never had before in my life. It was almost spiritual.

About an hour later I was called in again, to re-site a drip that had fallen out, and the brain surgeon extraordinaire came back to earth with a thud.

. . .

The second epiphany came a couple of years later. On hearing that I had passed the final exam and become a Fellow of the Royal College of Surgeons of England, my parents took me out for dinner in Manchester to celebrate, followed by a film. My dad, to whom I was by then very close, had already seen it, but he was raving about it so much he wanted me to see it, too. The film we went to see that night had a huge impact on me.

The Killing Fields is the story of the dreadful civil war in Cambodia between the government forces and the Communist Khmer Rouge. A Cambodian journalist and interpreter, Dith Pran, saves the life of American journalist Sydney Schanberg after they are arrested by the Khmer Rouge. Some time later at the French Embassy in Phnom Penh, when all the foreigners are being evacuated, an attempt is made to save Pran, too, as all educated Cambodians are being rounded up and killed in pursuit of the new regime's "Year Zero" policy of ethnic cleansing. The attempt to forge a Western passport fails, however, and Pran is sent to a concentration camp, where he feigns illiteracy. Upon his escape he finds the bodies of thousands of people who have been killed by the regime.

Eventually, after enduring many hardships, Dith Pran finds refuge in a Red Cross hospital on the Cambodian border with Thailand, and in a beautiful final scene is reunited with Sydney Schanberg. Schanberg asks for his forgiveness—although he had moved mountains to try to locate Pran after his evacuation and return to the US, writing hundreds of letters in an effort to trace his friend, he is forced to confront the fact that he'd also been pursuing his career and that leaving Pran in danger had been useful to him. "Nothing to forgive, Sydney," Pran says. "Nothing."

I found the film completely mesmerizing. I was an emotional wreck by the end of it, and in the car on the way home was quiet and absorbed in my own thoughts, still reeling at the intensity of what I'd seen. I remember Dad asking if I was all right.

The next day I went back and watched it again. The film lit a torch inside me. It vividly depicted the horrors of war—and I suppose I had always been interested in war, from my father's stories of Burma to my model-plane collection. But more than that, the film also depicted the incredible power of human love and friendship in the face of unimaginable adversity. And there were parallels with my experience. In one memorable scene Pran quietly but forcefully pleads with the brutal and fanatical Khmer Rouge to spare the lives of his Western colleagues—an example of the power of intervention, of stepping in to relieve and disperse pressure. There is even a scene set in a Phnom Penh hospital overrun with patients, where a surgeon has to deal with a shrapnel injury and complains about the lack of blood to infuse—I wanted to be that surgeon. I wanted to be a humanitarian doctor, in severe and stressful situations, using my knowledge to intervene and make a difference.

The film also spoke to me because I could relate to its depiction of innocent people being bullied, pushed around, or dismissed. I had been there, I knew what that was like, and felt the film was telling my story, too. It's always the weak who come off worst, and even more so in the modern era.

I began to feel a very strong sense of mission, an urge to work in war zones where my surgery could be put to good use in hospitals like the one in the film. What would I need for such a job? I'd need a fantastic breadth of knowledge in general surgery, which I was on the way to achieving. And I realized it would also be good to know a lot about vascular surgery, too: if I was to spend time in dangerous places I'd be seeing and dealing with a lot of injuries from bullets or bombs, and knowing how to clamp off blood vessels would be essential.

However, I couldn't just drop everything and go. From 1985 until 1992 I was on the path to becoming a consultant surgeon, and I knew I had to see that through before enjoying the freedom to pursue what I began to think of as a calling. My memory of *The Killing Fields* and the spark it had ignited still burned strong, but I felt if I left my job and went to work abroad at that time I would not have been trained to the high level of expertise required, and I worried I would never have been able to get back on track, as consultant jobs were few and far between.

I had to bide my time. I took a research post in Liverpool and ensured that the work was done in record time. I then became a senior registrar, also in Liverpool, and there followed a period of intense surgical activity and education. I now had the right to walk around the wards seeing the various cases, the different patients and their planned operations, and I could cherry-pick the ones I fancied and add them to my own list. I acquired a huge amount of experience in this way, expanding my toolkit of knowledge for the work that lay ahead.

Eventually, in 1992, seven years after I got my fellowship, this enthusiastic and idealistic young surgeon got his consultant post at Charing Cross Hospital in London. And then, toward the end of 1993, my chance came and it all began.

- 3 -
WELCOME TO SARAJEVO

In November 1993 a couple of colleagues from Charing Cross Hospital returned from a mission volunteering in the Balkans and were full of their experience. As part of my preparation for work overseas I'd already been on a two-week course with the British Red Cross to get my accreditation as a volunteer. But when I rang the International Committee of the Red Cross (ICRC) they told me I would have to go for six months, which would have meant letting down both my patients and my colleagues. My surgeon friends told me there was another way. Médecins Sans Frontières offered shorter placements—even of only two or three weeks. Provided MSF accepted you as a volunteer, it was up to you to decide how long to go for. So I rang MSF and then went for an interview with them. Even though I was now a consultant, I knew I might be committing career suicide by leaving my job even for a few weeks, but the lure to help had become irresistible.

The civil war in the former Yugoslavia had, by then, been raging for two years. Until the death of its "president for life," Josip Broz Tito, in 1980, the Socialist Federal Republic of Yugoslavia, a nation cobbled together across ethnic divides, had walked a delicate line between the planned economies of the USSR and its satellites and the liberalism of the West. Mostly it worked, and the constituent federal republics of Serbs, Croats, Bosnians, Slovenes, Kosovans, and others got along well enough. But the cracks began to appear a year after Tito's death, when Kosovo Albanians demanded their independence and then clashed with the Serbs.

The pot reached boiling point with the collapse of the Soviet Union a few years before. Multiparty elections brought the separatists to power, four of the republics declared independence, and the nationalists' arguments soon tipped into outright war—first in Slovenia and Croatia, then farther south in Bosnia and Herzegovina.

By the end of 1993 the country was deep into a brutal civil war. The Bosnian capital, Sarajevo, had been besieged and blockaded by the Bosnian Serb army since May 1992. For a cosmopolitan, outward-looking city, which only eight years earlier had hosted the Winter Olympics, the siege was unprecedentedly traumatic. And it was in Sarajevo that civil war turned from a violent conflict into a humanitarian disaster. The city's hospitals were understaffed, or even unstaffed, and innocent civilians were crying out for help.

Every night I watched the news from Sarajevo in a state of high anxiety, transfixed by the horror of what was happening. I could feel my heart pounding and my breathing getting faster. It was as if I were being physically drawn in. It felt very strange to have such a powerful physiological reaction to events happening far away, in a country I'd never visited, but a flame had been lit. I thought of how my father and his family had escaped the Japanese invasion of Burma and the suffering that had entailed. And I remembered my response to *The Killing Fields*, and the feeling of vocation it had sparked in me.

Perhaps this was the moment, and the place, to get involved?

Just before Christmas 1993 I packed some warm clothes and a sleeping bag and left my comfortable flat in Hammersmith to fly to Zagreb, the capital of Croatia, the newly independent country to the north of Bosnia and Herzegovina. I went straight to the MSF office, where I found a contingent of British plastic surgeons and a Belgian MSF staffer who briefed us on the logistics of our trip.

We pored over a map of the region while the MSF logistician drew on it to show us the front lines around Sarajevo, a city in a fairly narrow valley surrounded by hills and mountains, and told us that the Serbian army controlled the high ground to the south. He explained how to use the walkie-talkies we would be issued, and the correct radio terminology—something my flying experience had already prepared me for. Many things were new and strange, though: being told how and when to wear our flak jackets and helmets; the absolute ban on moving around independently; the different types of artillery being used on the city and the kinds of injuries we might expect; evacuation procedures; and the constant threat from snipers. It was all so surreal—I could hardly believe that I'd be in the middle of all this the following day.

There was much form-filling to be done, and disclaimers to be signed, and we were also told that we could back out, if we were having second thoughts and decided we didn't fancy going unarmed into one of the most dangerous places in the world. I certainly thought about it and had a sleepless night before we flew down to Sarajevo. But the sleeplessness was due as much to excitement as anxiety (and the cold—it was freezing). Also, I was a young man. I felt immortal.

Before we left Zagreb, we were issued our credit card–sized UNHCR passes—proof that we were working under the auspices of the United Nations High Commissioner for Refugees. The cards were more important than our national passports in some ways. As a civilian, you couldn't get in or out of Sarajevo without one. They changed hands for big money on the black market and the importance of keeping them safe was drilled into us.

After the briefing we had dinner, then went to our rooms to ponder the days ahead. Tossing and turning and hugging my sleeping bag around me for warmth, I wondered how I would cope with the challenge. I felt very confident in my abilities as a surgeon—much more so than when I'd been a junior hospital doctor, but was still prone to occasional bouts of self-doubt, even guilt, as I wondered about whether I was doing the right thing for a patient. What I didn't know—couldn't know—was how the environment would affect me. I knew there would be much less by way of equipment, but back then the phrase we would come to use for working in such places—"surgically austere environments"—meant nothing, and I was more worried about bombs and bullets than whether I would have access to a lot of high-tech equipment.

The phrase that came to mind—quite apposite, given the snow-covered hills around the city—was that I had committed to the slope. Like a skier at the top of a black run who can only continue once he's begun, I just had to go with it, try to dodge the patches of treacherous ice where I could, and make it to the bottom carrying myself—and hopefully some others—to safety.

. . .

The next morning we were driven back to the airport to board a Russian Ilyushin four-engined aircraft for the short flight to Sarajevo. There were a few other doctors on the plane but mostly it was filled with UN peacekeepers from Nigeria, in full battledress. The lighting inside the cabin changed from white to red as soon as we entered Bosnian airspace—the already heightened atmosphere on board becoming even more tense, almost disturbing in the eerie half-light, not least as we were instructed to put on our flak jackets and helmets.

As we approached Sarajevo we went into a shockingly sudden descent, practically a nosedive—the protocol was to descend as rapidly as possible and then circle tightly in a kind of corkscrew motion to make the plane more difficult to hit with a rocket or missile. The entire plane shook under the stress and I was certain we were going to crash, until at the very last second the nose pulled up sharply and the wheels touched down on the single landing strip in the shadow of Mount Igman.

Before we had a chance to catch our breath, the doors were flung open and someone shouted, "Get out! Get out!"—the plane could not stay on the runway for long, it was too dangerous—so we all grabbed our stuff and ran as fast as possible across the tarmac to what passed for arrivals. This was a shabby concrete building full of armed soldiers, who as soon as we came in made a dash for the plane we'd just left, which then promptly took off. It had spent less than ten minutes on the ground.

From the blown-out windows and shell-damaged airport buildings, with the control tower half-destroyed, it was clear we'd left the relative security of Zagreb behind. The desperate state of the city became more evident on the drive in: drab, postwar concrete apartment blocks and buildings, scarred by shells and fire; the municipal, Soviet-style architecture not improved by having great chunks missing nor the dank, freezing mist that seemed to hang over everything.

We were taken in an armored Land Rover first to the MSF office next to one of the city's hospitals, the Koševo Hospital. Here we had another briefing, but now to the tune of Sarajevo's soundtrack, the chatter of small-arms fire and the occasional *crump* of an artillery shell. The woman who received us looked terrible—drawn, haggard, devoid of humor, exhausted by stress. A psychiatrist by profession, she looked like she was nearing the end of the line. Her summary of the situation was stark, filled with warnings about the dangers from snipers and the various friends she'd known who had been killed. She seemed traumatized, perhaps literally shell-shocked. After the briefing I never saw her again.

My place of work was not to be the Koševo, though, but the larger state hospital in the city center—it became known as the "Swiss cheese" because it had so many holes in it. The state hospital was where the majority of casualties were first taken; Koševo was used more for reconstructive work on those patients for whom the immediate danger had passed.

My arrival should have provided some immediate respite to the people working there—I could see straightaway that the handful of surgeons, nurses, and anesthesiologists were exhausted and demoralized by the relentless stream of patients admitted hour by hour. But for some reason the two main surgeons seemed reluctant to let me loose on patients—I went straight to work but only as a glorified assistant. I got the impression they were suspicious because I looked young, and they had no idea how experienced I was or whether I was even competent. It's true that I had never seen injuries like the ones that were coming in every hour. I had witnessed the result of blunt-force trauma many times, but I was now seeing firsthand the effects of fragmentation injuries and high-velocity bullets. In modern mortars, bombs, and shells, the entire casing of the explosive is designed to fragment and fly off in all directions, causing terrible damage to soft human bodies.

Some of the injuries were too ghastly to describe here, but the main difference from my work in the UK was that so many casualties had missing body parts. Even in catastrophic car crashes, it is quite rare for someone to suffer traumatic amputation. But here it was routine. I was confronted for the first time with patients whose lives and deaths were synonymous with despair.

Another shock to the system was having people brought in, often in circumstances of high drama and emotion, who were clearly already dead. They would sometimes be accompanied by close family or friends who beseeched us to do all we could to save them, but we did not have the power of resurrection. All we could do was try to offer comfort to the living and make sure the body of their dead loved one was taken care of.

That first night I shivered again in my sleeping bag, but this time was kept awake by the sheer noise of the gunfire all around. It was constant, although the snipers tended to be quieter at night because they couldn't see their targets. But the shelling went on, and over time I would be able to distinguish between the sound of incoming fire from the Serbs and outgoing missiles being fired back at them. There was a subtle difference in pitch, and we became quite blasé about the sound of a rocket we knew was heading away from us.

My grunt work continued for the first two days—I was allowed to watch, and to fetch and carry and help, but the two incumbent surgeons did not allow me to operate on anyone. I began to feel frustrated by this and could not understand their attitude. I had come out to help them, hadn't I? Later, as I got to know the Bosnians better, I realized it wasn't personal, there was just an implicit understanding that volunteers like me had the choice to leave and go back to their warm, safe homes at any time, and that fact sometimes caused friction. They thought the same about journalists and the many other temporary visitors who regularly breezed in and out. On reflection, it would be a remarkable resident who did not consider me and my ilk to be "tourists"—an accusation that would be thrown at me later on in this mission.

On the third day, though, one of the surgeons didn't show up. In fact, he never appeared again. It remained a mystery whether he'd been killed, or if he'd somehow managed to escape. It was rumored he had gotten ahold of a UNHCR pass and used it as a ticket out.

I saw my opportunity and commandeered the free operating room as my own. I remember my first real patient very vividly—an elderly lady who looked to be in her mid-seventies. She had lost both legs, one above the knee and one below, and also an arm, all blown off by shrapnel. It was a horrendous trio of injuries, easily the worst I had seen at that point. She came in with her family, who were clamoring for action and solutions, and I just did not know what to do with her. She was conscious, but only just—she'd reached that antemortem point where unconsciousness is not far away, and is the prelude to death. The immediate response to trauma is pain, but after a while, or if the blood loss is too great, the body goes past the pain barrier and begins to shut down. It looked like she had reached this stage, and she lay there grunting softly with the sheer effort of staying alive.

My natural inclination was to dive in and start doing something, partly to be seen to be acting and partly because doing something is often easier than doing nothing. But was it the right call? She was old, and terribly injured. It was likely she would not survive a lengthy operation or a series of different procedures. We also had a finite amount of blood to give her. Should she get it? Or would tomorrow bring a more worthy recipient? Who was I to decide who was more worthy anyway? It might be better just to give her some morphine, take away any last pain she might be experiencing, and let her go gently.

I decided to operate, and began to debride her wounds: cleaning and cutting away dead tissue, removing bone fragments, and generally trying to move the odds in favor of the remaining healthy tissue. After about forty-five minutes of this, however, the anesthesiologist tapped me on the shoulder and said, "She's gone."

It was a depressing start. But such was the volume of casualties being brought in that there was little time to dwell on it, and before long the remaining staff came to realize that I did know what I was doing and could be left to my own devices. We began to work well together as a team, despite the strains and privations and danger. Most of them spoke a bit of English, and a few spoke very good English, but there would be occasional mix-ups: I remember thinking I was picking up a bit of Bosnian of my own when I'd hear a doctor call for what sounded like "Mackadoe! Mackadoe!" I wondered whether this was some comment on the stage of the operation reached, or perhaps a Bosnian swear word, until I realized that the cry "Mackadoe!" was always followed by a nurse handing over a pair of McIndoe scissors, named after the pioneering New Zealand surgeon Archibald McIndoe.

The bombs and bullets would usher people into our care, but in many ways the biggest problem was the temperature. The cold was biting in Sarajevo that winter. It seeped through my clothes and permeated my bones. It greatly affected the patients we treated, too. The operating room in which we were working was freezing. The water was cold when I washed my hands, my surgical gown was soon tatty and torn and we ran out of surgical masks, so I would watch my breath condensing in the cold air.

While uncomfortable for us, it was potentially deadly for the patients, some of whom would die from hypothermia before their wounds could kill them. Operating rooms need to be kept warm because when you open a patient's abdomen they lose precious heat very quickly. Temperature directly affects the outcome during surgery and if body temperature falls dramatically, the effects can be devastating. The body's enzymes stop working so that blood does not clot as easily; the heart does not beat properly and oxygen, our life source, is not used to best advantage. Organs begin to fail.

Most of the time the hospital generators worked well, and the thud-thud-thudding noise they made in the bowels of the building was clearly audible, but there was never enough diesel to keep them going and every now and then we were thrown into complete darkness, often in the middle of the night. When this happened, a man would come into the operating room with a wheelbarrow full of five or six car batteries. The batteries were then haphazardly wired up to a large lamp that the man held up, which became the operating light until the electricity flickered back to life. The lamp cast mediocre beams through the hazy chill of the room but was better than nothing.

One night about two weeks into the mission a youth of about sixteen was brought in. A large fragment had entered his abdomen. Sarajevo was at the time under particularly intense bombardment from tank shells, mortars, and rockets. The metal fragments from these projectiles produce similar injuries to those of bullets, but often larger and much more destructive. This young man was bleeding so badly that he had very low blood pressure and a high pulse rate, indicative of surgical shock. There were four of us in attendance: me, an anesthesiologist, a scrub nurse, and an assistant. The anesthesiologist and I discussed the option of surgery. We had a choice—operate and try to save his life, or not operate and watch him die. There were no other patients—it was about three in the morning—but we had very limited resources and it was freezing. We looked at the patient and nodded at each other, then took him into the operating room to do what was necessary to stop the bleeding. Once he was under anesthesia and being infused with the only pint of blood we had, I opened his abdomen.

The operation in which a surgeon examines all parts of the abdomen and pelvis is called a laparotomy. With your eyes and hands you examine all the solid organs in the abdomen, such as the spleen, liver, kidneys, and pancreas as well as all the hollow organs such as the stomach, small bowel, and large bowel down into the pelvis, which, in women, includes the bladder and the uterus. It also involves making decisions such as whether or not to expose large blood vessels such as the aorta, which takes oxygenated blood from the heart, and the inferior vena cava, which returns venous blood from the whole body to the heart.

After cleaning the abdomen, I made a long incision through the abdominal wall. As I made the incision longer, blood spilled in scarlet waves out of the patient's abdomen onto my hands. In the chill of the operating room, his blood felt hot on my cold hands.

The fragment had punctured his inferior vena cava. This was the first time I'd seen an injury to such a major vessel. The sliver of metal was still there and there was no option but to remove it, even though it was partially stemming the bleeding. My heart was pounding as I wondered whether I would be able to control the bleeding after removing it—I knew I'd need to pack the wound quickly. But as I gently removed the fragment a fountain of blood spurted out from the torn vessel. I grabbed a big gauze swab from the nurses' tray and pressed it onto the gushing area, and waited.

As I was thinking about what to do next, there was an enormous crash. The hospital had taken a direct hit. The whole building shook, I could feel my feet slip on the tiled floor that was slick with blood, and instantly I had the thought that the structure might collapse. And then, suddenly, within seconds of the impact, everything went black.

I don't mean just dark—it was absolutely pitch-black, with no sliver of light anywhere. The operating room was below ground level and had heavy doors shutting it off from the rest of the hospital. I couldn't see a thing: I could not see my patient, or my colleagues. I realized with a jolt that I couldn't hear them either, apart from general commotion outside the OR.

I was still pressing my swab onto the patient's inferior vena cava, and with my other hand felt the aorta, which is right next to it. As a vascular surgeon you can tell roughly what the blood pressure is just by palpating the aorta, and I knew that his was slipping. I squeezed his aorta with my fingers to try to occlude it, and thus maintain the blood pressure to his heart and brain. But I could feel his blood dripping from his abdomen onto my thighs and down to my ankles.

"Packs! Packs!" I shouted, hoping beyond hope there was still someone in there with me who could help.

Minutes passed, and an eerie calm settled on the room. I waited for the man to appear with the wheelbarrow and the lamp, but he did not come. I waited and waited, my fingers clasped around the boy's vena cava, but his pulse was getting weaker and weaker. In the cold silence I called out to the anesthesiologist, but there was no response. I called out to the nurse, to the assistant, but my voice just echoed in the darkness. The only thing I could sense was the tide of wetness as the boy's blood left his body; my shoes were squelching in it, my hand was cramping with the strain of holding on. I could feel his life slipping away.

"Hello! Hello! I need lights here! Anyone there?"

I called and called. And then, I knew the boy had died.

I was at a loss as to what to do, and just waited, the warm blood gradually becoming colder in that icy operating room. Some minutes later the lights began to flicker, and then came back on. I looked around the OR—of course, I'd drawn conclusions from the fact that no one answered my cries, but I was still shocked to see that I was all alone. My surgical team had fled to take cover. Without speaking to one another or saying anything to me, they had each decided the attack on the hospital was their cue to leave.

I looked down. It was like a slaughterhouse; the boy must have lost three or four liters of blood, much of which was on me. I stumbled out, shedding my gloves and gown, and felt a sense of utter despair. That boy should have survived. Maybe not the old lady, but the boy should definitely have survived. If the man with the wheelbarrow had come, if the lights had come back on sooner, if I'd had some help, we could have saved him.

I felt terribly let down. No one had said to me, "David, we're going, you've got to come, too"—they had just buggered off and left me there. I took off my sodden socks, and wandered in a daze down the hall, desperate for a kettle so I could boil some water to wash away the blood and warm my numb hands. I found the team in a sandbagged office down the hall—the anesthesiologist, the nurse, the assistant, even the wheelbarrow man. They just sat there. Not a word was spoken. There was no discussion. The body was simply taken away.

That boy's death, and in particular the way my colleagues reacted to the attack, changed me. Like many doctors and nurses I had always been very sympathetic and empathetic to my patients back home, taking bad outcomes very personally. But this experience taught me two things: first, I'd have to toughen up; second, I also had to take care of myself. Not just because there was no one else there who was going to do that for me, but because I wouldn't be helping anyone if I was dead.

It was like an initiation. I felt for the first time like a tiny cog in the vast machinery of war. My idealism was challenged, shaken; I was hardened by it, and better understood the intense pressure my colleagues had been under for so much longer than I had had to endure. The boy's death turned me into a person marked by war: it was the Sarajevo equivalent of a campaign medal, although not one to wear with pride. It manifested not so much in a tough exterior as a tough *interior*, a little place in my heart, or soul, that closed like a fist and iced over. It was arguably the first in a series of experiences that I bottled away, thinking I'd put them behind me, until a trip to Syria twenty years later.

The importance of self-preservation was brought home to me a couple more times on this first mission. One day I was asked to go to Zenica, about thirty miles away, to operate on a twelve-year-old boy who had an artillery shell fragment–wound to his neck. The tiny piece of metal had pierced the carotid artery and jugular vein and ended up in his larynx, where the vocal cords are situated. As a result the high-pressure carotid artery began pouring blood into the low-pressure jugular vein, putting significant strain on his heart, and he had developed a condition called high-output cardiac failure—basically, too much blood was being pumped into his heart and, after a while, it would fail. The connection, called a fistula, needed to be severed, and the carotid artery and jugular vein separated and repaired. I boarded a UN armored personnel carrier to travel through the Serbian lines to Zenica, which is in central Bosnia. At one of the checkpoints we had to go through, I remember the rather startling sight of a very beautiful Serbian woman, heavily made up and with immaculate red fingernails, who had an assault rifle slung over her shoulder and bandoliers of bullets to complete the look.

When we arrived the boy was in a bad state. He was taken into surgery and I duly operated on him. I was delighted with the results, and for good measure also removed the fragments of the bullet that had been lodged in his larynx. It was lifesaving surgery; he was going to be fine.

That evening, my colleague Darko and I decided to go for a walk in the city and we set out to try to find somewhere to eat. The cafe we chose was a pretty dismal place, with only a few chairs and no tables at street level, but there seemed to be a proper restaurant downstairs, so we headed down the narrow stairway in search of food.

There were maybe seven or eight tables dotted around, all of them occupied by hard-looking men in black leather jackets. They glared at us as we came in, and I noticed to my alarm that several had weapons lying on the table in front of them.

Rather than turning tail and heading straight out of there, we made our way over to one of the two free tables—there was one by the stairs and another across the room. I chose the table that was farther away but Darko wisely dragged me back to the one closer to the exit and we sat down. We ordered a couple of beers and some cold meats—there was no hot food. The atmosphere was tense, the men's demeanor aggressive, and I became extremely anxious. The whole restaurant seemed to be looking at us.

I tried to engage in some conversation, saying that I was a surgeon and had come to help and operate on a child in the hospital. One man—big, stocky, a bit drunk—stood up and said angrily that I was only there as a tourist, wanting to see what was going on. He came over to our table and demanded to see my UNHCR pass. Darko shot me a warning look, so I piped up, as calmly as I could, "I'm not sure I have it with me," all the while nervously fingering my pass in my pocket.

The man became very animated and raised his voice.

"You don't know what it's like!" he shouted. "You don't know what it's like to live in a war zone! I'm going to show you!"

And with that, he reached over for the switch, turned out the lights in the restaurant and started banging his chair on the floor and going around the room hammering his fists on the wall.

"This is what it's like!" he yelled, the chair going *bang bang bang* on the floor.

By now both Darko and I were seriously intimidated, certain that we would be attacked at any second, and I was damned if I was going to lose my precious pass—I wouldn't be able to get back to Sarajevo without it. We could just about make out a sliver of light coming from the door to the stairs. I shoved our table away from us and we bolted for the exit. As we ran up toward the street, we heard the sound of fighting breaking out behind us, great crashes as tables and chairs went over, and then gunshots. I didn't know whether they were shooting at us or not, and we didn't hang around to find out—we ran across a frozen football pitch nearby and headed back to our hotel. Later I discovered that there was indeed a shoot-out in the restaurant that evening, and several black marketeers had been killed.

That night we were lucky. Back in Sarajevo, the importance of not leaving the state hospital, of only traveling in armored vehicles, was drummed into us again and again. One day, foolishly, I broke these rules. It almost cost me my life.

I was enjoying the work so much, I felt I was doing some good, and I can't deny I was already bitten by the bug of adrenaline. The danger was a buzz. I felt that nothing could touch me. I was invincible.

So, when a patient needing reconstructive plastic surgery had to be transferred by ambulance from the state hospital to the Koševo Hospital, I asked the ambulance driver, a Bosnian guy who did the trip quite frequently, if he would take me with him so I could see the city from a different vantage point. He refused, quite rightly, knowing the protocols and also the dangers. But I persisted, and eventually persuaded him to let me tag along. I sat in the back, with the patient, who had a leg injury but was fully conscious, and a hospital porter sat up front with the driver. I wasn't even wearing my flak jacket.

Koševo Hospital is on a hill overlooking the city but far from the mountains that surround Sarajevo. The ambulance had just a large red cross on the front and the back, and I felt sure that this would stop the warring factions from targeting it. Not only that, but I knew that the Geneva Convention upholds the rights of health workers in areas of war and is supposed to provide protection from all sides.

The roads were wide and relatively clear, with odd bits of rubble and bomb damage to negotiate. Because the patient had severe wounds and fractures—and because it was a very icy day—it was decided we would drive slowly. It was normally only about an eight-minute drive, along a flat road and then uphill. We would have to negotiate a couple of checkpoints as well as the winding roads.

After leaving the state hospital, we traveled through the city center, the area most targeted by snipers. We had gone no more than five hundred yards before the ambulance came under attack.

The first thing I was aware of was the noise—a loud crack as the windshield went, followed instantly by the dull thud of bullets hitting someone's body. It was so quick, four bullets in rapid succession, but it felt like slow motion. My mouth was suddenly full of blood. I could feel it, taste it, it was in my eyes, too; I assumed I'd been hit but had no time to check before the driver, despite being shot in his left shoulder, threw the ambulance into reverse and careered backward to the safety of the hospital.

We screeched to a halt once we were safely inside the compound and I rushed to the other side of the ambulance and began to pull out the porter, who'd also been hit. I began to perform cardiopulmonary resuscitation but it was obvious he was dead: he'd been shot in the chest, neck, and face. Blood spattered the whole of the inside of the ambulance and I remembered that I needed to check myself, too—but despite all the blood, none of it was mine. Relieved, I then attended to the ambulance driver and, after a mug of hot, sweet tea, operated on him within an hour of his being shot.

It was terrifying, of course, and it took some time to process what had happened. It was a cauldron of emotions. At first, I felt guilty that I'd disobeyed instructions about leaving the hospital and stupidly put myself in such danger. I was worried about possible repercussions for my irresponsibility. And I felt guilty that the porter had died, although I later rationalized that he was going on this journey anyway; the fact that I was an extra passenger had not changed his fate.

There was also relief—relief that I'd survived, that I'd been shot at for the first time in my life but not been hit; relief that the sniper had killed the porter and not the driver, and as a result we were able to make our escape. And there was anger. We were in a clearly marked ambulance, emerging from the state hospital on medical business—it was outrageous that anyone should have targeted that vehicle. I felt righteously angry about it. Ever since that day, the cause of ensuring the sanctity and free passage of medical personnel in war zones has been very close to my heart, and not just for my own self-preservation.

But once the initial shock had faded, I had to confront another emotion that was more surprising, even a little disturbing. I felt elated, exhilarated, euphoric. I had never felt more alive; it was as if I had been reborn. I had come close to being killed, but that only made it more exciting. If I could cope with this, I thought, I could cope with *anything*.

Sarajevo was my first taste of this, and I knew I wanted more. It was a strange mix of altruism, wanting to help others, and pure selfishness—chasing the high of intervening to save lives, but also of living my own life closer to the edge. At home I lived alone—I had a few girlfriends, but nothing serious. It was a bit of a monastic existence and I had few material needs. But after Sarajevo I had to acknowledge that this was something I needed in my life. There was another world out there, one in which I could use my skills to change the outcomes of people's lives for the better—but also one in which I could experience the sheer thrill of being plunged into situations most people can't begin to imagine. The endorphin rush of hearing and feeling bullets and missiles whizz overhead was like nothing I'd encountered before, and everyday life seemed dull by comparison.

The BBC journalist Jeremy Bowen, who was in and out of Sarajevo at this time as well, captured this feeling very neatly in his memoir, *War Stories*:

> During the war the alternative – 'normal' life – seemed very tame. I had no desire whatsoever to be someone safe in London, commuting to work, knowing what I would be doing and when months in advance. In Sarajevo I felt free . . . That part of it, the feeling of living on the edge, was fun. The only constraint was making a mistake that could get you wounded or killed, which was straightforward in a way that I liked.

I'm told it's not uncommon for war correspondents to feel this way—another veteran reporter of many conflicts, Anthony Loyd, called his own memoir *My War Gone By, I Miss It So*. I suppose there are parallels between our roles—we're both noncombatants, going into extreme places as neutrals trying to do some good, whether saving lives or telling the world about an atrocity.

And, as is sometimes the case for journalists, it was very difficult not to get involved in the reality of the experience for the people on the ground, whose lives were being torn apart. I felt for them keenly. The citizens of Sarajevo were lovely people who had not harmed anyone yet were being harmed. I did not know them or their past lives, but they were very vulnerable and it is the vulnerability of human life that—when it is stripped down to its basics—makes us all the same.

Most of the civilians I encountered in Sarajevo were warm, generous people. They went out of their way to make me food and to give me gifts and presents when things went well. They also understood when I couldn't help them. And they reminded me so much of my Welsh family. They were surrounded by the green, green grass of their home, but at the same time they were encircled by mortar fire, tracer bullets, and bombs. But despite the language barrier I felt I totally understood who they were and what they were feeling. It was like being at home again.

I came back to London a different person, knowing that I could really change the lives of people in dreadful circumstances. But I came back angry, questioning how people could do this to one another. It seemed to me that there was a very fine line between those who have power and use it wisely, for the greater good, and those who attempt to destroy all competitors.

But to be granted that God-given ability to help people in their time of need was the most joyous gift that I could ever have imagined. I knew it would be part of my life from then on.

-4-
DAMAGE CONTROL

I had learned so much in Sarajevo—not least just how much I still had to learn. I returned to the UK both humbled and energized by the experience, determined to improve and expand my surgical toolkit before going anywhere else. From the end of 1994 I took up the three positions in the NHS that I still hold today, at St. Mary's, the Royal Marsden, and Chelsea and Westminster. One of the many disciplines I knew I'd need to get better at was obstetrics, which covers pregnancy, childbirth, and the postnatal care of both mother and baby. I had been interested in obstetrics as a medical student, and at one stage considered specializing in it before settling on general surgery. My time in Sarajevo had shown me a little of the extraordinary stress being in a war zone put on expectant mothers. Not only were they already anxious about the experience of giving birth, perhaps for the first time, but also the world they were bringing their child into was dangerous and uncertain. Over the years I came to appreciate that being able to perform a safe emergency Cesarean section or manage postpartum bleeding was one of the most useful, even essential, skills for a humanitarian surgeon.

But I didn't learn how to do a Cesarean in the safety of a London teaching hospital. I learned the procedure in Kabul, the capital of Afghanistan, while working for the International Committee of the Red Cross. It was 1996, two years after my trip to Bosnia, and I had used the intervening time to try to hone my skills while settling in to my new jobs, eager for the next overseas opportunity. The 1990s would come to be seen as a relatively peaceful decade around the world—the Cold War was over, and the "War on Terror" yet to begin—but there were areas of conflict nevertheless. And Afghanistan was a place where conflict seemed to be a semi-permanent state.

I went at an interesting time in the country's history. Since the fall of the Soviet-supported Communist leader Mohammad Najibullah in 1992, Kabul had been under the control of various warring factions. Infighting among the mujahideen produced many casualties, who kept us busy, but the real struggle for control of Kabul took place in September 1996. I was the surgeon on call in the ICRC field hospital when the Taliban rolled in and captured the city after intense house-to-house fighting including shelling, rockets, and gunfire. We were all worried that the situation would spin out of control. The Taliban's reputation for brutality preceded them, and although their arrival was greeted with singing in the streets, we feared they would treat us as infidels and kill us. Najibullah was still living in Kabul, holed up in the UN compound. The Taliban overran the complex, captured him, and summarily executed him by hanging him from a lamppost in the city center.

Before my arrival I had been on many ICRC courses, including their pre-deployment course, the war-surgery course in Geneva, and a residential British Red Cross course for a week near Guildford. The organization's founding principles—humanity, impartiality, neutrality, independence, voluntary services, unity, and universality—were drummed into me. Sitting in a quiet classroom, it's easy to gloss over how profound such ideas are, but out in the field they are the essential commandments that allow the ICRC to work almost anywhere in the world.

At the hospital that day, I definitely had a feeling of impending doom as I heard the Taliban getting closer and closer, but was reassured by the calmness of the project manager, who had been working hard to secure our safety as well as the security of the hospital. We looked after war-wounded but we also dealt with all the surgical procedures you'd expect in a district general hospital anywhere in the world: obstructed hernias, perforated stomach ulcers, bowel and urinary problems. We also took care of the health of pregnant women and their unborn babies, everything relating to what I believe is nature's greatest miracle: childbirth.

In austere environments, it's very common for women in obstructed labor to require a Cesarean. I had never been taught how to perform the procedure; it was, for me, a "holy grail" operation that I'd always wanted to learn. In most Red Cross hospitals there is a roster between two surgeons—one who normally works full-time with the ICRC and is the senior surgeon, and another who is usually an expat on sabbatical from his hospital at home. The senior surgeon in Kabul, Yuca, had worked for the ICRC for years, and I both admired and respected him. He could turn his hand to anything.

On my second day in the hospital, he asked me if I could do a C-section. Of course, I had to say no, and I will never forget his eyes rolling to the back of his head.

"So you must understand that I like my sleep," he said, "and usually the midwives will call for a C-section at 0400."

Within a few hours my chance had come—a woman in her early twenties in obstructed labor. She went into surgery and was given a spinal anesthesia in double-quick time.

There are two ways of opening the abdomen for a Cesarean section—a midline incision or a lower transverse cut called a Pfannenstiel incision. This is the incision of choice, as the wound heals much better than a midline incision.

"You do the operation," Yuca said. He didn't even scrub up, just stood over my shoulder and barked instructions on where and how. *Bloody hell,* I thought as I made the incision just above the pubis.

"Spread the rectus muscles, pull harder, pull harder! You British are weak."

I had not seen a C-section since being a medical student, and this was a baptism of fire.

"Cut the peritoneum here," he said, grabbing a long pair of forceps and pointing at the place, "push the bladder down. Now get your scalpel and make the cut into the uterus."

The lower segment of the uterus comprises the stretched uterine muscles and the upper part of the cervix. It tends to be less muscular and, when cut into, does not bleed as much as the very muscular uterus, which, by full term, has a blood supply of 600ml per minute.

"Cut, cut! Go on, cut!"

I cut into the uterus and my heart leapt as blood and amniotic fluid poured out in vast quantities. My scrub nurse removed the retractor and I pushed my right hand in and felt the baby's head.

"Flex it, flex it!" Yuca shouted. *What does he mean?* I wondered, but now was not the time to ask. Suddenly the head popped out, and with that the shoulder. I put my fingers under the armpits and with a push from my assistant, out shot the baby.

I was mesmerized. It was incredible. My heart was pumping with excitement and wonder, so much so that I forgot to clamp the umbilical cord and was instead trying to show the baby to her mother. The scrub nurse clamped and cut the cord for me, and we waited for contraction of the uterus to deliver the placenta.

"Good, now sew it up," I heard as Yuca turned on his heels and walked away, shouting over his shoulder, "and now you don't have to call me!"

It was a wonderful operation. I had helped create one life and saved another. I would never be able to do this at home in London, but here in Kabul it was an operation I was mandated to do, and I did every C-section for the remaining weeks of my mission.

After the Taliban took control, they renamed the country the Islamic Emirate of Afghanistan, and imposed strict Sharia law. When I returned there in early 2001, this time working in the Taliban's spiritual birthplace of Kandahar, I was able to see for myself the impact this had on the country and its people.

It was like going back to medieval times. Women were confined to their homes, children were not allowed out and were forbidden to play with toys, especially of Western origin. Education was banned apart from studying the Koran, and innocent pleasures like kite-flying or playing music were also banned as they took children away from the study of Islam. Women had to cover themselves from head to toe in sky-blue burkas, with crochet mesh covering even their eyes, and men were not allowed to shave their beards.

The hospital where I worked, Mirwais Hospital, had five wards, three for men and two for women. Men and children were not allowed to visit their wives or mothers, no matter how ill they were. Even if they were dying, they would have to die on their own. The only men allowed into the ward were the surgeons, of which there were seven local Afghans and the ICRC expat. Once, during a ward round, I was taken to see a patient by one of the expat nurses. We were followed by some of the local nurses, dressed in their all-enveloping burkas. As we stood by the bed one of them nudged me. I looked down as she lifted the hem of her burka to show me a flash of her ankle. She was wearing fishnet tights, perhaps even stockings. I don't think she did this because she liked me, I think it was an act of defiance against the terrible rule of the Taliban.

I could see Mirwais Hospital from my first-floor bedroom in the mission building where we were staying. There was another prominent building visible, too, less than a mile away, a large compound notable for its sandbagged walls and heavy security. I wondered what it was for. One night we were all shaken awake by a huge explosion nearby. I threw myself out of the bed onto the floor for cover. A security guard ran up to see if I was OK, but it seemed to be a one-off as there were no more explosions. In the morning I found out that the blast had come from a cruise missile that had been sent in to destroy the compound I had been looking at in the distance. The house was still standing; it had missed. Someone at the hospital told me that the house was the residence of the al-Qaeda leader Osama bin Laden, who was living in Kandahar at the time. I treated one of his wives for a fibroid problem, and the ICRC surgeon before me had treated bin Laden himself for kidney stones. Apparently, he was due to come back for a follow-up—but he never came to his appointment with me. It's an odd feeling to look back on this near-brush with a man who, only months later, would cause such devastation, with all the chaos and conflict that would ensue. *If only I'd known*, I would joke—but of course I didn't know, and there's nothing I could have done anyway.

Although we worked in the hospital, the Taliban ruled it. Every day, a Taliban policeman wearing a large black turban stood inside the entrance to the operating room. He was there to give consent for us to operate on patients, and make sure we were not contravening any of the strict religious codes imposed by the regime. We had to ask him if he would allow us to operate on this or that patient, knowing he had no medical knowledge whatsoever and probably couldn't read or write either. A simple wave of his hand would submit patients to lifesaving surgery or sentence them to death.

We had four operating tables going at the same time, and I was always amazed by the stoicism of the Afghan children who came in. If they were having elective operations, they would walk in hand-in-hand with their father, often having to witness other operations going on, sometimes with gruesome glimpses of another patient's anatomy or body parts lying in buckets. Unfazed, they just walked casually past and without a fuss got on the operating table, ready for their surgery.

The maternity ward was downstairs, run by an expat midwife along with several local nurses whom she had trained to perform normal deliveries. One day while I was operating, the midwife ran up to say they had successfully delivered a baby boy but the mother was bleeding very heavily and they were having terrible trouble stopping it. As they had tried to remove the placenta it had torn, and the patient was rapidly becoming shocked and needed urgent attention.

Through our interpreter, I asked the Taliban policeman whether she could go in for surgery immediately, expecting it to be a formality. To my amazement, he shook his head. I couldn't believe that he was denying not only the mother her chance of life, but also the little baby boy his mother. We began to plead with him, but despite our entreaties the interpreter eventually conveyed that the policeman had made his decision, and that in his view it was only right that the mother should die. The expat midwife then ran to fetch the head nurse, a formidable woman called Ingrid. We had to do something fast as the patient was bleeding out: Martin, a German expat anesthesiologist, ran upstairs from the maternity suite to say that if we didn't operate on her soon she would die.

Ignoring the Taliban policeman, Ingrid and I ran out of the hospital, jumped into a car and told the driver to take us to Mullah Omar, the Taliban leader. We drove down to the center of the town near a very beautiful mosque covered in blue mosaic. I was amazed that the cleric agreed to see us, but Ingrid was very forceful and would not take no for an answer. I stood there with her as she raised her voice to one of the most feared people in the world. His manner was serene, almost statesmanlike, and there was no perceptible malice as he stared at me with his one eye. Just to get rid of us, I think, he agreed to our request for permission to operate and we sped back to the hospital.

How the news had spread to the Taliban policeman in the hospital I will never know, but he signaled his assent with a curt nod of his head and we rushed the patient up to the operating room. By this time she was as white as a ghost, with desperately low blood pressure and a rapid pulse. She was cold and sweaty and it wouldn't be long before her low blood pressure caused her liver and kidneys to fail, which would mean a slow death even if we successfully managed to perform the immediate lifesaving surgery.

I looked at her and wondered what to do. There are various techniques a surgeon can use in this situation to stop internal bleeding, such as packing the uterus with swabs, pressing on the uterus to try to compress it, or inserting a medical balloon and inflating it. She had just had her sixth child and her body was in shock, and I wasn't sure if any of these techniques was going to be effective. I decided to operate.

Martin quickly put her to sleep. He began to transfuse the only bag of blood that we had for her. I wasn't sure what I was going to do, so I opened her abdomen with a long midline incision. I had heard about a technique whereby you can put sutures into the uterus to compress it and that was what I was considering as I entered her abdomen. However, I found that her uterus was huge and tense and very thick-walled. Even though she had had the drugs to contract the uterus, they hadn't worked. The midwife reminded me that the placenta tore and could not be removed. Then it hit me: she must have had a condition called placenta accreta where the placenta erodes into the uterus. I had to think quickly; she needed a hysterectomy. I had never performed this operation before but, having been trained in colorectal surgery felt I knew my way around the pelvis pretty well.

I carefully placed clamps on the side of the uterus and divided the ligaments and fallopian tubes, carefully working my way down, ligating the various blood vessels supplying the uterus until I could feel the cervix. The blood vessels surrounding the uterus were enormous, the size of my finger; if I hit one of them it would cause massive and overwhelming hemorrhage and, with the small amount of blood that we had to spare, would certainly have been fatal. Very carefully and with intense trepidation, under the watchful eye of the Taliban minder, I removed the uterus just above the cervix. There must have been at least three liters of blood in there. Amazingly, the patient survived, but it was touch and go for the next few days. To this day, I cannot understand the mind-set of that Taliban policeman and after the operation I viewed him with utter disdain. Where does it say in the Koran that you can play God?

I had to be careful, though, because he was very dangerous and also very vindictive. I had got to know one of the male nurses in surgery, a man called Mohammed who was an extremely good scrub nurse. One day Mohammed didn't show up for work, and I asked where he was. This was greeted with silence from the other nurses and doctors, and a quick and surreptitious look at the policeman. Mohammed, I learned, had cut his beard because he wanted it to fit under his surgical mask to reduce the risk of infection. But the policeman felt that this was against Islamic teaching and he had ordered Mohammed to be locked inside a shipping container in the middle of the street for twenty-four hours.

This was a notorious punishment for people caught doing supposedly anti-Islamic acts. Mohammed told me after his release that there were at least fifty people in there with him, with no access to food and water and no toilet facilities, with excrement and urine flooding the floor. It was totally dark inside and the only light cast was by the occasional opening of the door to let somebody in or out. The temperature inside the shipping container was around 120 degrees Fahrenheit. It was a horrendous way to treat people.

Because we worked for an aid agency, we were permitted to go to the city's football stadium to witness the enforcement of Sharia law, Taliban-style. Idiotically, I went along one day only to witness terrible and unforgettable acts of barbarism: women being stoned to death after being buried up to their necks in sand; women being placed beside a wall they had built with their bare hands and killed after a truck was driven at the wall at high speed. There were also revenge killings, where the victim's relatives were allowed to shoot and kill the supposed perpetrator. I felt like a spectator at some brutal entertainment from ancient Rome and was reminded of a bullfight I'd once seen in Provence, where I had been appalled by the killing of those magnificent animals. But this was far, far worse.

The images of what I saw all those years ago still flash through my head sometimes—so easy to view, so hard to shake. I often wonder now why I went. I think it was because I simply didn't believe what I'd been told about what went on there. I also couldn't believe that what purported to be legal in Sharia law was nothing more than outright murder and torture. I was astonished and sickened by the cruelty that one human being could bring to bear on another, and it filled me with revulsion. The football stadium was full of people watching and I wondered what they all felt. Were they completely inured to it? Or just curious?

I also wondered what it must be like for the people receiving the worst of the sentences that the court handed down. Minor offenses like stealing a loaf of bread would lead to terrible punishments. I watched from a distance as people queued to have their hands or feet amputated with a single swipe of a machete. Many of these poor amputees made their way to the outpatients' department at the hospital with their hand or foot in a plastic bag and then asked me to sew it back on. Nowadays, with all the microscopic instruments available, it is possible to do this sort of surgery in specialized units. But it was out of the question in Kandahar at this time, and all I could do was try to refashion the stumps of the forearm or lower leg into proper covered amputations. At least these unfortunate people were given back their amputated body parts for them to bury according to Islamic law.

Six months later the world entered a new era, with the attacks on New York and the Pentagon on September 11, 2001. Like everyone, I was shocked and horrified by these events, and I found it bizarre to think that I'd been working among people who shared the terrorists' ideology just months before.

Almost immediately Afghanistan was plunged into further conflict, as the governments of George W. Bush and Tony Blair assembled their coalition to hunt down bin Laden, the mastermind behind the attacks. Bush issued an ultimatum to the Taliban government in Kabul to hand bin Laden over, and when they refused to comply he launched Operation Enduring Freedom, with British and other allies, to oust the Taliban. Kabul fell in mid-November, but the al-Qaeda leader evaded capture, and was assumed to have slipped across the border into Pakistan.

Meanwhile, as is well-documented, influential neoconservative figures within the Bush administration were attracted by the opportunity 9/11 presented to move against a longstanding adversary of the United States, the Iraqi dictator Saddam Hussein. Despite there being no evidence of Iraqi involvement in 9/11, and indeed Saddam being a known critic of al-Qaeda, the War on Terror swept him up, too. Airstrikes began in March 2003, with Baghdad falling a month later. Saddam's regime was over but Bush's claim of "mission accomplished," as expressed in a banner behind him as he made a speech on board the USS *Abraham Lincoln* in May, proved horribly hubristic. The country was already sliding into a hugely destructive and violent insurgency, with the number of casualties, both military and civilian, *after* the supposed victory over Saddam vastly exceeding those incurred during the invasion.

In the initial invasion of Iraq, British forces had been instrumental in taking the southern port city of Basra, home to around a million people. After the collapse of the regime the British remained in control and would stay there for another four years. Throughout this period I volunteered regularly for MSF and the ICRC, going repeatedly to different African countries. But, of course, I followed events in the Middle East closely, and in 2006 decided to join the Royal Auxiliary Air Force as a volunteer reservist. In part this was maybe a way of living out my boyhood fantasy of becoming a pilot, but I'd also had an inspiring conversation with my colleague and friend Pete Matthew, who was already in the Royal Auxiliary Air Force with 612 Squadron at Royal Air Force Leuchars, and who suggested that seeing how things worked in the military would be a great way to learn new techniques and improve my trauma portfolio.

Despite my model-making, my love of flying, and fascination with war stories as a boy, I was actually a little uncomfortable with the idea of working for the armed forces. It seemed to go against the grain of my humanitarian work, but I knew that it would give me access to all sorts of courses and meetings that would otherwise be closed to me. My real motive was to learn, and I would then be able to use that knowledge and share it with my colleagues in the field. So I signed up, was given the rank of Squadron Leader (the lowest rank offered to qualified surgeons), and was told I'd have the opportunity to work in Basra in 2007.

I expected to face a great deal of danger in Iraq, and indeed sustained a nasty gash to my leg after falling off a Snatch Land Rover and impaling myself on a metal mudguard which had been twisted and deformed by a bomb blast—my very own shrapnel injury. This was nothing compared to one of the junior doctors I attended to after he'd effectively been blown up by an incoming rocket. He had multiple shrapnel wounds on his face and, such is the black humor of military medics, he ended up being nicknamed Dr. Peppered.

However, I had not anticipated that I would experience a brush with death in genteel Chelsea the week before I left. The hospital I work in there has a revolving door, which is stimulated by a sensor. Half the door rotates outward and the other half inward. One day there were about twenty people held in one half of the door while a boy of about twelve was standing under the sensor on the other side, laughing his head off with a couple of his mates. I saw what was going on and pulled the boy away, so that people could get into the hospital. He fell onto the floor and before I knew what was happening, he took out a boxcutter and jabbed it into my neck, in full view of all the people there. A woman screamed and I stood stock still, waiting for the pain that never came—the blade, luckily, was still retracted into the body of the knife. If it had been open it would have gone straight through my carotid artery and jugular vein, and I certainly would have died. The police were called and scoured the surrounding streets for the boy after they all bolted, but he got away.

I arrived in Basra as the British presence in the city was winding down, although not because there was nothing to do. The British forces had pulled back to the contingency operating base at Basra airport, and our field hospital was a tented structure on the base. The army was still doing sorties into Basra using Warrior vehicles and the casualties from roadside bombs were becoming intolerable. In addition to the risk posed by IEDs on the roads, there were rockets and mortars raining down every day on the operating base. Over a period of six weeks that summer, on the base alone there were fourteen killed and at least sixty wounded. The sirens would go off, indicating an imminent attack, and everyone on the base would quickly put on their helmets and body armor and crash to the floor, hiding beneath or behind any object that could take the impact of a piece of fragment from an exploding missile.

It was a strange position to be in, almost fetal, hands underneath your body with your head buried in the helmet and your legs and feet tucked in as closely as possible. As the alarms went off a strange feeling would come over me—everyone could hear the sound of mortars landing and sometimes they were extremely close, but I always felt that one would never land near me or cause me any harm. It was like, *This is happening, but it won't happen to me.* Defending us was an anti-missile system called Phalanx. This was a Navy-designed array comprising a matrix of sensor-activated guns to intercept incoming fire. It locked on to any incoming rocket or mortar that was fired into the air base. The sound was like a firecracker going off but lasted for much longer, and reportedly took out nearly three-quarters of all incoming rockets.

In the operating room we were often on the floor, with the patient still on the operating table, while missiles were raining down. It was just pure luck that we survived the day. The surgical team was as exposed as everyone else to this onslaught, but it had the benefit of bonding us together. In fact, one of the things that made the mission enjoyable was the camaraderie I experienced as part of a military medical team. On aid-agency missions, I was often the only surgeon in whatever facility I found myself in, and sometimes the only Brit, which could be lonely and sometimes led to tensions.

Here, though, there were no such cultural differences, and what I really enjoyed about the military setting was that everybody was trained to the same level. We all went through pre-deployment training, including weapons-handling and learning how to deal with an ambush. We also understood the authority of commands during an attack. The battlefield medicine training involves an advanced trauma life-support course and the management of casualties during firefights. Later, the defense medical service would set up a military operational surgical training course, and all surgeons and surgical staff went through it prior to deploying to Afghanistan. But this was not available before I went to Iraq in 2007. The surgical support at the Basra air base consisted of a general surgeon, an orthopedic surgeon, anesthesiologists, an operating team of nurses, and a nursing team to manage the wards. We also had junior doctors, radiographers, and physical therapists.

We were all kept very busy, and our field hospital operating room sometimes looked like the back of a butcher's shop. Many times we operated in helmets and body armor as rockets pounded the base.

One terrible day encapsulated the intensity of the mission. I had moved rooms as my air-conditioning unit had broken down, and my new room was next to an accommodation block near an area called the Trenchard Lines. This was where many of the RAF ground crew stayed. That day, July 19, 2007, I was for some reason playing with my camera in my room when the alarm sirens went off. I still have the picture of the moment when a large mortar shell landed on the accommodation block next door. On that day, there had already been at least half a dozen indirect-fire attacks and luckily nobody had been injured, so the hospital was fairly quiet. But the moment the mortar landed I knew that there would be huge casualties. Senior Aircraftsmen Matthew Caulwell, Peter McFerran, and Christopher Dunsmore were all killed immediately, and many others were injured. My pager went off and I hurried to the emergency room.

Quickly the casualties began to come in. One man had a significant wound to his left arm; all the bones around his elbow were destroyed, as was soft tissue including muscles, nerves, and arteries. He was resuscitated and the team's orthopedic surgeon and I managed his case jointly. In war, the orthopedic surgeon manages the bones and the general surgeon the soft tissue. I was confident I could repair the blood vessels. The airman had lost a significant proportion of the muscles of his arm but I was sure I could still put the oxygenated blood back into his arm via an arterial bypass graft.

His main problem was that the nerves were severely damaged and his bones largely destroyed. I wanted to salvage the arm but the orthopedic surgeon wanted to amputate. There were pros and cons for both options, and it was probably six of one and half a dozen of the other. However, a surgeon always wants to do his best for the patient and sometimes we take a radically different view from that of our colleagues. A standoff ensued, and the atmosphere quickly became explosive. We had a furious argument over the operating table on the correct management of the case. It went on for an extraordinarily long time while the anesthesiologists grew more and more anxious; the patient had lost a lot of blood.

Eventually, the orthopedic surgeon won the argument and we amputated. In the end it probably was the right course of action, as all the nerves were severed and would have required nerve grafting with success far from guaranteed—he would probably have had long-term pain and been left with a functionless forearm and hand. As it was, Senior Aircraftsman Jon-Allan Butterworth went on to win three silver medals for cycling in the 2012 London Paralympics and a gold medal in the 2016 games in Rio and has raised thousands of dollars for charity.

Despite occasional differences of opinion, practicing emergency medicine in a military setting was revelatory. War has long been recognized as a driver for technological progress, as combatant governments plow resources and expertise into trying to give themselves the edge over their enemy. But there are other, more benign side-effects, too, and one that had a major impact was the development of what became known as "damage control" surgery during the wars in Iraq and Afghanistan.

The more I learn about the human body, the more amazed I am about how it works. Since the whole purpose of blood is to transport oxygen to our vital organs, significant blood loss means that we lose the capacity to transfer oxygen in sufficient amounts to those organs, which then begin to shut down. All the cells in our body require oxygen to generate heat—this is called aerobic respiration. Lack of oxygen means the cells cannot produce energy and so our body temperature falls; another by-product is lactic acid, which, in turn, increases the acidity of our blood. All the chemical reactions in our body require a normal temperature and neutral acidity. Therefore the consequences of losing a lot of blood are that we become cold and bleed more, because the clotting enzymes don't work. Having a cold circulation with high acidity also affects the heart, which begins to fail and does not pump adequately, and so even less oxygen is delivered to the organs.

When a casualty arrives with a gunshot or fragmentation wound, we now know that the most important thing to do is to try to reverse the effects of lack of oxygen to the tissues. The combination of hypothermia (cold), coagulopathy (impaired ability of the blood to clot), and acidosis (raised acidity) is called the "trauma triad of death." If you do not reverse these conditions as rapidly as possible then the situation will become intolerable and the patient will almost certainly die.

Studies have shown that around 30 percent of casualties who have lost a lot of blood by the time they arrive at a field hospital will already be hypothermic and coagulopathic. It is therefore important to recognize that these patients will already be entering the trauma triad of death. "Damage-control" surgery is, in effect, a temporizing measure to reverse the effect of hypothermia, coagulopathy, and acidosis. The source of the bleeding is found and quickly stopped, while plastic tubes called shunts reestablish blood flow to the arms and legs if arteries are damaged. The patient is on the operating table for a much shorter initial time, and can then be taken to the intensive care unit to be warmed up. When the patient is more stable, they can be brought back to the operating room to undergo whatever definitive surgery is necessary, such as reestablishing the blood flow using vein grafts or performing bowel reconstruction, all of which takes time.

During the Iraq and Afghan wars, the principles of damage control surgery were taken to a higher level, with constant hands-on experience leading to continuous refinements and improvements. A major advance was the development of damage control resuscitation, which involves replacing lost blood with preheated blood, thus minimizing the effects of cold and poor clotting. These techniques have now been adopted by all the major trauma centers in the developed world.

In Camp Bastion in Afghanistan, where I went to work in the summer of 2010 during Operation Herrick, we had over a thousand cases of major trauma over an eight-week period. But because everybody worked as a team and knew exactly what their role was, including performing damage control surgery and damage control resuscitation, the hospital there had amazing results: 98 percent of all those who were shot or who had major injuries from IEDs survived. It was a remarkable achievement, as some of the casualties had terrible wounds such as the complete loss of both legs and, in some cases, also an arm, the so-called triple amputation.

A case I dealt with halfway through my tour encapsulates how good the care at Camp Bastion really was. Throughout the war there were teams of civilian contract workers all over the place, employed by companies that supplied the military with sophisticated electrical equipment. One of these contract workers had been shot in the abdomen near Lashkargah, about thirty miles from Camp Bastion. The call went out to the medical emergency response team (MERT), and a Chinook helicopter was dispatched. The crew comprised two pilots in the front and, in the back, a consultant anesthesiologist, a consultant emergency physician, and several nurses, with an RAF Regiment gun crew providing firepower.

The worker had been hit by a Taliban sniper's bullet. When the crew got to him, he was in a terrible state. During the transfer back to the camp he suffered a cardiac arrest and needed liters of blood. We received the call "op vampire," which meant they were giving resuscitative blood en route to the hospital. These calls usually meant that the patient would take a direct right turn into surgery on arrival rather than going through the CT scanner. I was ready and waiting with my team of anesthesiologists, surgical assistants, and a whole host of backup support, all ready to swing into action. The doors of the operating room flew open and the man, still being given external cardiac massage as well as rapid infusion, was carried in. We had lots of blood lined up and everything was set to give him the best possible chance of survival.

He had been shot just above the navel. The emergency physician who was on the helicopter had done a secondary survey and now shouted to me that there was also an exit wound just to the right of the spine. This was a high-velocity, high-energy gunshot wound through and through. There was no time to stop and take in any more information. He needed the operation now. I made a long laparotomy incision from just below the sternum to the pubis. Liters of blood spewed from his abdomen all over me and onto the floor. The infusers were pouring in blood via large IVs in his arms and there was also one in his neck. Usually in this situation the correct surgical procedure is to pack the abdomen as quickly as possible to try to staunch the hemorrhage. I had no time to do this—I had to turn off the faucet as rapidly as possible. I had two options: either open up the chest and put a clamp on the distal thoracic aorta, or delve down as rapidly as I could to feel the aorta with my fingers just below the diaphragm and press it against the lower thoracic vertebra, like pinching the end of a hose. Once I'd got into the abdomen, I chose the latter technique. I called out to my assistant,

Squadron Leader David O'Reilly, to pack the abdomen while I squeezed the aorta. He did so as best he could but we both noticed that where the liver should be was a mess. It had been completely destroyed by the bullet.

The effect of a high-velocity, high-energy gunshot wound is well known. The physics of ballistics is a vast topic, and whole institutions have grown up researching the effects. A low-energy 9mm pistol bullet gives up its energy fairly rapidly on hitting a target—if it hits muscle, for example, it will cause some cutting and laceration of the tissue. But a high-velocity, high-energy bullet from a semi-automatic rifle causes massive damage. Einstein's theory of relativity can be applied to all sorts of things, including the transference of kinetic energy from a bullet to someone's body. Einstein's insight was to show that kinetic energy is equal to half the mass times the velocity squared—the heavier the bullet, the more energy is transferred into the organ that it hits. If the velocity of the bullet is doubled, then the energy released is quadrupled.

And when a high-energy bullet from, say, a sniper's rifle hits a target, then the bullet tends to tumble inside the body. It tumbles because its center of gravity is well behind the point, and as it slows down it becomes unstable. This tumbling effect dissipates huge amounts of energy, so if it hits an organ of high resistance such as the liver, which is enclosed in a layer of connective tissue called Glisson's capsule, then it can literally blow the liver apart. This is what had happened to our patient.

Under my fingers the aorta was beginning to pulse, and I could feel the man's blood pressure improving. I had been squeezing his aorta for around forty-five minutes and I was relieved and grateful when the anesthesiologist told me that both blood pressure and heartbeat had regulated. The thumb and first finger of my right hand had become numb with the pressure and extremely painful. I got David to press down on the aorta for me until I could clamp it off completely. It was only then that we could see the full extent of the damage. We put clamps on the remaining bits of liver that were hanging on to the inferior vena cava and very rapidly stitched up all the holes.

After about four hours our patient was still with us. His heart was beating well and his lungs were able to oxygenate his body, but he had no liver, and for good measure his kidneys had also stopped working. He went to the intensive care unit and it was decided, I think for the first time in military medical history, to try hemodialysis. The dialysis machine was gathering dust in a cabinet and the engineers had to work on it through the night to get it up and running. Once it was working properly, it was able to eliminate the toxins that the liver and kidneys usually take care of.

The next morning I went to see the patient in the ICU. I was amazed that he was doing so well. His blood pressure was normal, although he needed medication to stimulate the heart's contractions, and he was no longer bleeding. From the moment the worker had been shot his chances of survival were very slim. But thanks to the amazing teamwork and all the equipment and expertise available, he survived an incident that ordinarily would have had a near 100 percent mortality rate. Instead, when he had recovered sufficiently, he was transferred to the UK and went on the list for a liver transplant.

The trauma unit at Camp Bastion was then regarded, rightly in my view, as the best trauma unit in the world. I am proud to have been part of it, and thrilled that these techniques are now filtering out beyond the military world and helping the poor civilians caught in the crosshairs of combat.

- 5 -
FLYING IN

I don't know how many lives I have saved over the course of my career: it's a question I am often asked but never know quite how to answer. There are the very memorable or dramatic interventions, some of which I describe in this book, where I know for certain that if I hadn't done what I did, the patient would have died. But does that mean that someone else would not have stepped in if I hadn't been there? And, when working in a conflict zone, I very often never discover how my patients fare in the longer term. Have I really saved someone's life if the postoperative care isn't available, or good enough, and they succumb to some infection or other a few days later?

Maybe such questions are best left to philosophers. For the surgeon faced with someone in need, the instinct to fix that person is powerful. And, of course, it is felt even more keenly if the person in front of you is someone you love. I hadn't been able to save my mother, and it was horribly tempting to indulge in the "what if" of identifying her problem earlier. Nor was I able to stem the inexorable advance of my father's illness, although we gave it a good try.

Toward the end of 2003 he had a recurrence of the colon cancer that had first been diagnosed the previous year. Mum and Dad were both living with me full-time. Mum used to go back to Carmarthen for a bit of a break, leaving me with the tricky task of managing Dad's care at home while doing my job at the hospital. I geared everything around making sure he was comfortable and well hydrated. In the mornings, to relieve his bowel obstruction, I would insert a nasogastric tube and aspirate around a liter of fluid from his stomach. I came home from work at lunchtime and put a drip on him to make sure he had enough fluids.

He told me that he had no wish to leave me or my mother, and wanted to live as long as he could. My colleagues at the Chelsea and Westminster Hospital were fantastic, bending over backward to help me through this difficult period. Dr. Neil Soni, one of the intensive-care anesthesiologists, even placed a central line in my father's neck so that he could be fed without having to eat. The dietetic department at the hospital were also wonderful, and every couple of days I would pick up a full three-liter feed from them. I even used to take my father's blood tests and top him up with blood at home every now and again.

But it was clear he was dying, and this added to the stress of what was already a miserable period, because I had been accused of negligence by the family of a patient who had died, and the case had gone to the General Medical Council. It was as if the Sword of Damocles was hanging over my head, ready to drop at any moment. The negligence case was particularly upsetting because I had liked the patient a lot. I was sure that the reasons for her death were unrelated to anything I had done and I couldn't understand why everyone seemed to be gunning for me. I became very disheartened, and seriously considered giving up surgery altogether.

Flying has always been one of my passions, from my fascination with Airfix models as a little boy to joining the RAF cadets at school. Inspired by Ray Roberts, I had got my glider pilot's license at sixteen and my private pilot's license when I was seventeen. Flying was an important part of my life, and when I became a consultant, I decided I wanted to get my commercial pilot's license, too. I bought a little Cessna and spent as much free time as I could racking up the hours I needed. Eventually, I also earned my flying instructor rating, an airline transport pilot's license, and a helicopter license, too.

Having gone along with my father's wishes as a teenager, when I'd agreed not to join the Royal Navy and fly helicopters but become a doctor instead, it was perhaps ironic that toward the end of his life I was considering packing in surgery and making flying my new career.

I applied for a job with Astreus Airlines, had an interview with them, and was accepted for a flight test. The test was at Gatwick Airport, in the simulator, flying a Boeing 737 from one waypoint to another and also landing the airplane on my own. When the day came, I spent the morning being briefed on the 737's systems, its instruments, and exactly what I was supposed to be doing, and then after lunch I went for the test itself. With both my commercial license and instrument rating under my belt, I felt fairly confident about the challenge of flying on instruments. In hindsight this was naive, if not arrogant—I should have done a bit more homework and perhaps practiced on the simulator at home using my computer. But life was so busy, and the days passed by so quickly, that it didn't occur to me.

I sat in the cockpit of the 737 simulator and realized with horror that I couldn't read the instrument panel at all with the glasses I was wearing. I have always worn fairly thick glasses to do close-up work. As we age, we all become presbyopic, or long-sighted, but I had inherited a gene from my dad that meant this happened to both of us much earlier than usual. I could certainly look out into the distance through the cockpit window onto the runway with the glasses that I had on, but the instruments were a blur. Also, the lights in the simulator were turned down, which reduced my vision even further.

There were two examiners in the back of the simulator, notebooks and papers at the ready. I asked if I could go to my bag and get a different pair of glasses. So there I was, taking this crucial test, wearing two pairs of glasses, one so I could see out of the cockpit window and the other so I could read the instruments. And even that didn't quite work—the reading glasses only helped if I leaned forward and got right up close to the instrument panel. The test lasted half an hour and I must have looked very peculiar bobbing backward and forward on the pilot seat trying to control an aircraft at 2,000 feet, while going from one navigational beacon to another and then landing back into Gatwick. When it was over the examiners were silent, apart from saying that they had never before seen a pilot with two pairs of glasses on the end of his nose. I was sure it was a complete bust and felt very disappointed as I drove home.

Amazingly, though, three weeks later I had a letter from the airline to say that I had passed the test, and they were offering me a further interview for a job as a first officer. I had the opportunity of a new life as a full-time airline pilot—but I panicked. I had several phone conversations with them before going to the interview, trying to work out whether it might be possible to somehow combine surgery with flying. The job they were offering me was on a roster, with two weeks on and two weeks off, and seemed like the perfect solution.

The problem was, I would need to be away for a month, learning how to fly a 737. But I could not leave my father. I couldn't even suggest when I might be able to take up their offer, because I didn't know how long my father would live. I had to say no.

At about the same time, and to my enormous relief, the negligence case against me was dropped. I knew I had not done anything wrong but still it was very distressing to be accused and then have to wait while the legal process unfolded. I think my father fought his illness just so he could be with me until a resolution was reached. It became his whole reason for staying alive. Within three days of the case being dismissed, he was dead.

The end came quickly over one weekend in the spring of 2004. My mother stayed with me for a month after my father's death before I drove her back to Wales. I spent a while there with her but was then offered another mission, this time to the Ivory Coast with MSF. The journey to Africa gave me more time to think about what I wanted to do with the rest of my life. The General Medical Council decision had lifted a weight from me, and flirting with the airline job had made me realize that giving up surgery completely was not an option I could countenance. My NHS job provided me with stability, so I could continue with my humanitarian work.

The flying dream was far from over, though. I did later find a role that enabled me to indulge my love of regular sorties, and took an occasional job with an aviation company called Hamlin Jet flying out of Luton Airport. I had learned to fly a Learjet 45 by going on a three-week course in Tucson, Arizona, coming home with the Learjet rating on both my American and British licenses. On weekends when I was not on call, I would swap my surgical scrubs for a proper pilot's uniform with stripes on it and I would metamorphose into a Learjet first officer. I spent about ten years with Hamlin, having a really good time—a dream come true for the teenager who had badly wanted to be an airline pilot.

The Learjet 45 is like a very complicated computer. It has so many banks of buttons it is sometimes easy to forget which ones to press. To remain at one's best as a pilot requires continual practice. You also need to enjoy what you're doing and not be too stressed, otherwise you make mistakes. Unfortunately, going off on humanitarian missions for months on end sometimes made me rather a liability in the cockpit. I realized my moment had come when I had just returned from a demanding mission in Afghanistan, and the ops manager called Hamlin Jet and asked whether I was available to act as copilot on a flight to Geneva from Heathrow.

The Learjet was based in Luton, so late one Friday night, only just come back from Camp Bastion, I finished off a busy clinic and headed up the M1. The traffic was terrible and I arrived harassed and hassled. The captain was furious. Planning the route, checking the fuel, and so on were my responsibility, but because I was so late the captain had had to do them himself. I arrived within about ten minutes of our takeoff slot from Luton to Heathrow.

On a commercial flight the captain has ultimate responsibility but the job is divided between the captain and first officer into "pilot flying" and "pilot non-flying." The pilot flying takes off and lands and monitors all the flight instruments and autopilot in response to any emergencies. The pilot non-flying performs all the other duties, such as radio communication with the air traffic controllers, and relays that information to the pilot and supports the pilot throughout the flight. We agreed that I would be pilot flying from Luton to Heathrow and he would be pilot flying from Heathrow to Geneva. The flight time from Luton to Heathrow in a Learjet is very short, not much more than ten minutes. It is busy airspace, though; there is a lot to do and it is very stressful.

We took off from Luton and all was going well until we were about 200 feet above runway 27 Left at Heathrow. Landing a modern jet is really flying by the numbers: the most important things a pilot has to do are maintaining the glide slope using the instruments in the cockpit and keeping the correct speed all the way down to the runway. Any deviation of either would have compromised the landing.

I turned off the autopilot, put my left hand on the throttles and my right hand on the control column, and tried my best to maintain both parameters. Having not flown for a while, and being under a lot of stress, I misjudged and dipped the airplane below the glide slope. Our speed increased to around 132 knots, when it should have been around 127. I raised the nose of the aircraft but the speed did not reduce, so I then reduced the throttle but ended up going below the optimum speed.

The captain by this time was shouting in my ear "Speed! Speed!" My heart lurched and I could see this was going to end badly. We crossed the threshold of the runway far too fast, which meant we did not touch down until about halfway along it. In my headphones I could hear a Qantas Airbus A340 talking to air traffic control saying he could see a Learjet on the runway in front of him, and that he did not have enough time to land behind it so would probably have to do a go-around. My captain went puce as I finally touched down but then promptly missed my turnoff. He grabbed the controls and somehow got us off the runway as the Airbus landed only a short distance behind us.

As we approached the stand, all was not well in the cockpit.

The captain told me he was going to get the passengers, threw me the flight plan for our journey to Geneva, and stormed off. I had about thirty minutes to get everything organized for the next leg. As pilot non-flying this time, I had to enter the flight plan in the flight-management computer, talk to the Heathrow director and the ground air traffic controller, and start one engine in preparation for taxi. I tapped the plan into the computer and spoke to the director to get our departure details. I could see the captain coming back with our passengers. When I received the departure details I began tapping them into the flight-management computer on the console between the two pilot seats. But every time I put the flight plan into one computer, the screens went blank on the computers and on the main navigation instrument screen.

As the captain came closer and closer, I grew more and more stressed. Thinking that I had to do something, I started one engine for the taxi. It should have been easy; it only required the press of a button. But I somehow managed to drop all my papers on the floor between my feet. By the time he made it into the cockpit, nothing was in the computers, nothing was on the navigation screens, and the information about our takeoff slot was on the floor.

The captain looked at me and shook his head. I knew he had blown a fuse, but it was obvious he was trying to remain calm for the passengers' sake. But when he realized I hadn't entered the information on the flight management computer, his rage became even worse, and with a cataclysmic expletive he entered the flight plan himself, pressed a few buttons, and we continued our taxi to 27 Right. I was also useless on the radio; I had become a gibbering wreck. Our flight to Geneva progressed in total silence, a silence that continued in the taxi to the hotel after our arrival. It was time to hang up my professional airline hat.

I have continued to fly, though. I've made a lot of good friends while flying and it remains a wonderful release after the intensity of the operating room. Floating above the clouds and diving down between them at will, seeing the splendor and beauty of the British countryside is simply dazzling. I hold a flying instructor rating having been taught by the best pilot I have ever known, Peter Godwin, and have taught many of my colleagues, some of them from their first experience of flight to sending them off solo and shaking their hands when they passed their private pilot's exam.

In 2007, when a group of British doctors were planning to climb Mount Everest, I was the pilot who ferried them around while they were training in Scotland and Norway. I also went to Canada with them for an ice-climbing course a year before their ascent. I was only the flying taxi-driver, but they still taught me how to rock-climb using ropes and gear and also how to ice-climb using crampons and ice axes. Just before their departure, a couple of team members wanted to do a bit more climbing in the Lake District. My very good friend Mark Cox, an anesthesiologist, was discussing this with me while we were operating, and I said it would give me great pleasure to take him up to Ullswater by helicopter. He was going to stay in the Leeming House Hotel, just by the side of the lake. We Googled it and found that I could land the helicopter in front of the hotel. What could be more perfect?

I hired a helicopter and Mark and his friend Roger arrived at Denham Airfield with a heavy load of climbing gear. The weather was beautiful, with blue skies forecast all the way. A takeoff slot of four o'clock in the afternoon would get us there in plenty of time for a leisurely dinner. I did a quick calculation and found that we were very close to our maximum takeoff weight, with all the equipment and full fuel in the tanks.

Once we had loaded up, I started the helicopter and made the call for departure. I pulled on the collective lever to gain some lift on the rotor blades and found that we really didn't have any. Eventually, with full takeoff power we finally got into the air. The journey was really wonderful—flying over the hills and mountains of the Lake District was an incredible spectacle. As we approached Ullswater I could see the hotel in the distance.

We were at about 3,000 feet when I started my descent. Usually in a helicopter it is better to put as much air into the rotor blades as possible, so you come down like a bird using its wings as brakes. I reduced the power and put the helicopter into a sixty-knot descent, aiming directly at the field. With about 1,000 feet to go, however, I noticed that there were a lot of sheep in the field below us—one of the rules is that you must land at least 500 feet away from any animal or person. So I chose another field, which was actually closer to the hotel, but my flightpath was such that I had to go around and do another approach. I banked the helicopter and we flew over the lake to gain height for the second approach.

It was trickier than the first—and there was another problem in that, rather than flying into the wind, I instead had a bit of a tailwind. I was also too high, so I steepened my approach. Now I was going a little bit too fast, so I slowed my speed. I was concentrating on the field and only too late did I realize that I was coming in far too quickly. I pulled up the lever to gain more lift but this only made the situation worse—we started to descend much more rapidly. Now I was in really big trouble. "Oh shit!" I blurted out.

I had about a hundred feet to play with, and forty of those were taken up by the hotel, getting larger and larger in front of me. The helicopter began buffeting and shaking and it looked like we would crash into the hotel's roof. Beyond the hotel there was a steep hill. The low rotor horn started to go off, telling me that we were about to stall; its high-pitched beeping didn't help. I looked at my speed, which was now around twenty knots. I had entered into a situation called a "vortex ring," in which the helicopter loses all lift while in a steep descent. In this situation, the tips of the rotor blade produce a downwash which forces the helicopter toward the ground rather than increasing lift. I had less than a second to react. I needed to increase the rotor revs because otherwise the blades would stall and we would crash immediately. I had to increase the power—but that meant pushing the lever down, making us descend further. I also had to increase my speed. Turning left was not an option because there was a tree in the way and turning right might send us into the roof of the hotel, but there was no other option. My margin of error was now all of twenty feet—I was sure we were going to crash, but banked to the right and cleared the roof by about two feet, coming down the side of the hotel toward the parking lot. With this maneuver I reached about fifty knots, and with the low rotor horn still blaring we were at least now producing a little bit more lift. Inch by inch we started to go up. I had nowhere to go but toward the hill behind the hotel. I had no idea if we had enough power to get over it, or if we'd simply crash into the side of it. There was nothing I could do. I didn't want to touch the controls as we were still going up, and I didn't want to do anything to stop that, but did we have enough lift to climb over?

The hill loomed larger and larger, and sheep started running in all directions below us. Then I noticed a power line going across the hill. Usually, in training, you are taught to fly over the top of a telephone pole, to ensure you don't hit the wire. I did not have enough lift or power to do that, so I had to aim for the middle of the power line between two posts, which was the lowest part of the cable above the ground. The skids of the helicopter lay a good couple of feet below the main body of the machine, and as I approached the line I wasn't sure I had enough clearance. I visualized snagging it with the skids and flipping over—there was nothing I could do apart from keep going. I closed my eyes for a brief second as we approached the cable. How we cleared it I will never know. It must have been by inches.

I aborted the hotel landing and flew on to Carlisle Airport, realizing I had had a very close shave. Mark, Roger, and I shared a taxi to the hotel and along the way I called my flying instructor, David Neiman, to confess. I received a good telling-off, all the while pressing the phone to my ear so that Mark couldn't hear.

Clearly, it was best not to try to combine flying and surgery, but events sometimes caused them to overlap. One late October afternoon I had been doing some flying at Biggin Hill Airport, south of London. As I was taxiing along in my little single-engine Cessna, one of my colleagues at Chelsea and Westminster called to say that a young woman had been brought in with a severe liver injury. She had been riding pillion on a motorcycle that had crashed on Battersea Bridge, and was bleeding to death on the operating table. Could I come in?

It usually takes around two hours to get from Biggin Hill to central London by car. I told them I was sitting in a plane, which I'd have to park first, and that I couldn't get there for an hour and a half at least. The consultant needed me sooner than that: "David, she will be dead in the next half hour, I can't control the bleeding."

As I was taxiing to the stand, I had one ear in my headphones focused on air traffic control and the other ear on my cell, phoning 999, the British emergency line. I got through to the operator and she asked what my emergency was.

"I'm a surgeon at Chelsea and Westminster Hospital. I'm at Biggin Hill Airport in Kent, but I need to get to that hospital within half an hour otherwise a girl is going to die."

She put me through to the police at Biggin Hill, who told me to wait outside the airport gate—a police car would be there within five minutes. Sure enough one arrived and I got in the back. The driver told me to sit in the middle and hold on to the two straps that were dangling from the roof. It was undoubtedly the most exhilarating fourteen minutes of driving I have ever experienced—with our blue lights flashing, we went through every red light we met and drove on the wrong side of the road into oncoming traffic, all the while with the policeman in the passenger seat shouting directions to the driver from a road map. It was absolutely incredible. We arrived at the hospital within twenty-five minutes of my receiving the call in the Cessna. As I dashed out of the car the policemen called after me to call them and let them know the outcome.

I quickly changed into my scrubs. As I walked into the operating room there must have been twenty people in there, including three anesthesiologists, three surgeons, and two scrub nurses. Many instrument sets had been opened up and there was blood on the floor and tension in the air. I went up to Tim Allen-Mersh, one of the surgeons. "Dave," he said, "thank God you're here, I'm losing her." I quickly looked at the monitors, which showed that the girl's blood pressure was 40 systolic—normally it should be around 120. I could see that the right lobe of her liver was in pieces and that there was a huge tear in the diaphragm. She was bleeding profusely from one of her hepatic veins, one that was really difficult to get to.

Generally, when confronted with a bleeding liver, you attempt to stem the hemorrhage by pressure and compression, in the hope that you can reestablish its anatomy. However, in this case there was no liver to compress, although the left lobe was still intact. I tried to pack the top end of the liver where the injury was, but blood was just sluicing out. Two anesthesiologists were squeezing blood in with their hands with another four or five units of blood next to them. The only option was to turn off the inflow to the liver and also to clamp the inferior vena cava, the main vein that takes blood to the heart. I put my finger into an anatomical space called the foramen of Winslow, behind the portal vein and hepatic artery, which is the inflow to the liver, and placed an arterial clamp across them. I then quickly dissected the inferior vena cava and put a clamp on that, too. Before doing this, I yelled to the anesthesiologists that they really needed to put as much blood into the intravenous lines as they could. These lines had been inserted into the subclavian veins, which drain blood from the head and neck and upper limbs; I was going to turn off the lower venous inflow from the abdomen and lower limbs. As I did this, I asked the nurse for a 3-0 Prolene suture and some surgical felt, which I could use to buttress my stitches.

I had one shot at getting it right. If I was unsuccessful and the bleeding hepatic vein tore even further, she would bleed to death. I had the luxury of many assistants by this time, and positioned everyone's hands where I wanted them. So much surgery in this type of situation relies on getting it right the first time. The needle holder has to be the correct length, the tips have to hold the needle firmly, and the needle must be positioned accurately in its jaws before even attempting to stitch. In desperate situations, even though you might inwardly be shaking with tension, it is critical that you remain calm. I have seen surgeons tremble so much that they were unable to place the stitch. To get the best out of the team around you, you need to radiate serenity. The whole team responds to the lead taken by the operating surgeon. Being aggressive does not help. You are one member of a team who are all working together to achieve the same goal. The person holding the needle is just one small part of the bigger picture.

Sometimes, other injuries can even help. The tear in the girl's diaphragm was so big that it exposed the whole of the inferior vena cava just before it entered the heart, and one of my assistants was able to press on it with their fingers, which allowed me to see the hole without too much bleeding. I was also lucky that the patient was young: the tissues were elastic enough that they did not tear when I put the suture through. The bleeding stopped with one suture. I couldn't believe my luck. I slowly took the clamps off the inferior vena cava, the portal vein, and the hepatic artery and started to reperfuse the liver with oxygenated blood. There were many bleeding points that I needed to contend with. She had lost so much blood by this time that she was getting cold and the blood wasn't clotting properly, and I needed to get her off the table as quickly as I could so that we could warm her up in the intensive care unit.

I made sure that all other organs were being perfused and packed the abdomen as much as I safely could. The diaphragm was in tatters, but—following the rules of damage control surgery—I decided that could be repaired another day. The packs went into her chest. There was nothing more I could do. A few hours later she was well enough to be transported to the intensive care unit. I left the hospital at around 11:00 p.m. and took a taxi back to Biggin Hill. On the way I called the Metropolitan Police to thank them, because—so far, at least—the girl's life had been saved. I got back to my flat at around two in the morning, and there were no missed calls on my phone, which was always a good sign.

The next day I learned that they had been struggling with her all night, but on the whole, she was stable, with a good urine output, which is probably the best indication that her circulation, and therefore her blood pressure, was strong enough to ensure that her kidneys were working. I left her in ICU for a further forty-eight hours before taking her back to the operating room. I always seemed to miss her relatives, as I was doing other things. When I took out the packs I could see that the intensive-care doctors had done a fine job of getting her coagulation back to normal, warming her up, and keeping her oxygen levels high. I was able to take all the packs out and close the diaphragm with a special mesh. She was going to make it.

The following day I went back to the ICU and finally met the girl's parents. They were obviously in shock because her boyfriend, who had been driving the motorcycle, had been killed. I spoke to them gently and told them that their daughter was going to be fine. Her mother remarked that they had been so lucky: Professor Allen-Mersh was such a wonderful man. I smiled, agreed, and walked away.

There have been many times when I have been called in to help colleagues in trouble. I even nicknamed my bicycle "Thunderbird," as it was always taking me around on international rescue missions. It has given me great pleasure throughout my career to be able to drop in and out of operations like this, and to have been able to help fellow surgeons in times of crisis. It's a bit like my humanitarian work. The patients don't know who I am—I just fly in and fly out, having hopefully made them better.

I've not yet had another crazy but unforgettable drive through the streets of south London in a police car, but there was one in Yemen a couple of years later that generated almost as great an adrenaline rush.

I was working in a small hospital in a town called Razeh in the Saada governorate in the north of Yemen. The civil war there had been going since 2004 when the dissident Shia cleric Hussein Badreddin al-Houthi launched an uprising against the Yemeni government. Most of the fighting took place in Saada. Above us, we could hear the sound of warplanes on their daily bombing runs from their base in Sana'a, to the south.

The taxi-drivers in Yemen were lunatics. It was only really safe to take a taxi first thing in the morning, because after mid-morning they'd all be high as kites on *khat*, a leaf that when chewed releases chemicals similar to amphetamines. They'd take a wad of *khat* and tuck it into their cheek, chewing on it for hours on end. By lunchtime their driving was completely erratic and twice as fast as it had been earlier.

Yemen was pretty scary. There is a real weapons culture and it is a highly chauvinistic society. Almost everyone carries a gun, usually quite openly, including all the nurses who came to work with us every morning. Weapons are more than tools for self-defense, hunting, or waging war in Yemen; they are status symbols and visible proof of social standing, manhood, and wealth. As is the *jambiya*, the curved knife that is worn on the front of their dress—the more elaborate the *jambiya*, the more prominent the man.

But sometimes the weapons they carried were more than symbols. I was told one story of a father whose hospitalized daughter began suffering powerful muscle spasms and facial contortions. She was experiencing something called hypocalcemic tetany, but unfortunately the father's diagnosis was that she had become possessed by the devil, and it was obviously her doctor's fault. The father's response was to start shooting up the hospital with a .50-caliber weapon, blasting away at anything he could see. The doctor escaped only by jumping out of a first-floor window, breaking both his legs in the process.

Before the drive up to Razeh, which was high in the mountains, we all had to fill in "proof of life" forms that were then sent back to the ICRC headquarters in Geneva. These forms are designed to ask very specific and personal questions to which only you will know the answer, so if we were abducted and a message got through to our captors, a single question could confirm our identity and that we were still alive.

The journey to the north took around ten hours, and we passed through some of the most beautiful countryside and architecture I've ever seen—extraordinary mud-brick buildings etched with white filigree and crowned with either stained-glass windows or translucent alabaster windows called *gammariya*. Some of them are up to fifty stories high. One of the reasons that Yemen is blessed with these amazing structures is that it had been ruled by xenophobic imams who, for decades, had shut out all foreign influence. Sana'a's beautiful old city is now recognized by UNESCO as a World Heritage site.

Razeh is also a beautiful place. But getting there was perilous. I clung to the straps for the entire journey, as I had in the back of that police car. The sound of gunfire could be heard all the time and people came to our little hospital having been shot either by forces from the south that were infiltrating the countryside or from stray bullets being fired by the locals, whose aim was far from perfect.

No one opened up in the hospital with a .50 caliber while I was there, but neither was it exactly safe. One day I was operating with my trusty nurse, Youssef. I was working on a patient's femoral vein when there appeared a crack in the window, as if a bird had crashed into it. I immediately looked to my right and saw what appeared to be a bullet hole in the glass. Youssef looked at me, and then fell to the floor. A bullet had hit him in the abdomen; it had missed me by about six inches.

He lay on the floor under the operating table, groaning in pain. The rest of us ducked for cover, leaving the patient on the table. We shimmied over to Youssef and quickly undressed him. There was a single gunshot wound just below his chest. What were we to do? Were we under attack?

I wondered if I could operate on him on the floor. There was only one room to operate in and I had my headlamp on, so I didn't really need any major operating lights. Youssef was becoming shocked and pale and needed an operation soon, or he would die. I realized I had to get him on the table. Two people came into the OR and took the patient off the table, bundling him outside to the corridor, still intubated.

We quickly shoved the operating table over to the side of the room that was shielded by one of the walls, and which, therefore, seemed relatively safe from further attack through the window. If it was a general assault on the hospital, though, continuing to operate for another two hours or so would put us all in jeopardy. Maybe the right thing was to evacuate and take cover? The consensus, however, was that whatever else was happening, we had to save Youssef.

The anesthesiologist took some blood from him and quickly identified his blood group. We didn't have any blood in that group, but the day before there had been a blood drive with many people offering blood in return for money. As a result we had quite a few units of O-negative, which can be used universally. The anesthesiologist quickly put Youssef to sleep and I counted out ten large packs of the swabs I would need. When I made the first incision, around a liter of blood poured out. The bullet had traversed the right lobe of the liver with an entry and exit point just below the rib cage. But Youssef was lucky, it had not hit any major blood vessel.

This time, I was able to press the liver together to try to obliterate the hole it was bleeding from. There is another way of stopping bleeding from the liver, although I'd never tried it until now. I passed a urinary catheter along the track of the bullet, then cut the middle finger off a surgical glove and tied it onto the catheter, so that when water was poured down the catheter it inflated the finger of the glove like a balloon, exerting pressure on the bleeding blood vessels. It was a success, and I left it in place along with some packs around his liver. Youssef was brought back to the operating room forty-eight hours later to complete the surgery. I told him to rest and take at least a month off work, but he was back standing next to me ten days later.

Another close shave, and perhaps another of my nine lives gone. Why did I keep putting myself in these situations? Once they've had a brush with real danger, I guess some people shiver and think, *Never again*, while others think, *Wow!* I had discovered I was definitely in the latter camp. I can't deny I get a kick out of taking the controls of a plane or a helicopter, or performing surgery in a war zone; the risk is part of the appeal. And it is undeniably addictive. It is a physiological reaction, as well as an emotional one. The trick is knowing when to stop, as any ex-junkie will tell you.

- 6 -
UNDER AFRICAN SKIES

Two years after my first trip to Afghanistan, I volunteered to go to Sierra Leone with MSF. A country of about six million people on the west coast of Africa, this former British colony had been beset by a succession of violent coups and counter-coups since achieving its independence in 1961. Its vast diamond resources, and the struggle to control them, were major factors in the civil war that had been raging across Sierra Leone since 1991. When I arrived there in early 1998, I found myself working in the Connaught Hospital in Freetown, the capital city, where the fighting was out of control. As in Kabul in 1996, various armed factions were fighting among themselves, and the civilian population was really suffering. There were sporadic attempts made by the government to reassert itself, but government support was always quashed violently by the militias, most prominently the Revolutionary United Front (RUF).

Initially the RUF had been welcomed by the Sierra Leoneans, who resented a Freetown elite seen as corrupt and were persuaded by the RUF's promises of free education, healthcare, and a fair distribution of the diamond revenues. However, the power of the gun soon turned them from a force for good to a force for evil. I had thought the Taliban were bad, but Sierra Leone was another shocking insight into man's inhumanity to man. The RUF began attacking civilians, carrying out mass amputations as a terror tactic. What makes people do this to one another? It must in part be the exercise of power without control or fear of retribution. Once people start blindly obeying irrational authority and conforming in both mentality and dress, it becomes easier to dehumanize your enemies.

Gangs armed with machetes paraded around the streets, hacking off the hands of government supporters. I spent several weeks simply refashioning amputations of the upper limbs of children as young as three, as well as elderly men and women. It was depressing to see the mindless violence meted out, but it was also repetitive and distressing work. Hundreds and hundreds of civilians were maimed by these out-of-control groups of children and young adults, who had been cajoled into taking up arms by their vindictive leaders.

I gave my camera to one of the local staff and asked him to go out one day and take a short video of what was going on. He came back with footage that still makes me shudder. A member of the opposition had been strapped to the hood of a vehicle like an animal and was being brought back to be shown off to one of the RUF generals. The boy driving the vehicle wore a chain around his neck. Hanging from the chain, like an amulet, was a severed finger. Just outside the hospital you could also see a man walking around with a machete held menacingly high, seemingly on drugs, with no fear of the authorities. With no fear of anything, in fact. It was one of the most lawless places I've ever been.

A year after my tour of duty in Freetown, I volunteered to work in Monrovia, the capital city of Liberia, the neighboring country to the south. Rebels from Sierra Leone had spilled over the border and were engaged in intense fighting with government troops. In this conflict, most of the rebels were high on drugs a lot of the time, and would often prance around naked to show how "manly" they were. Of the many wounded rebels and soldiers arriving at the hospital it was easy to tell which was which—they'd either be naked or wearing a ragged military outfit. Both sides seemed to be possessed of a crazed bloodlust, and many also wore small trinkets and trophies around their necks in the belief that this would ward off their enemies' bullets.

Our hospital was often on the front line, with incoming fire passing through windows and hitting the walls around us almost every day. Amazingly, though, not a single person who was working in the hospital was wounded while I was there.

We tend in the West to talk about Africa as if it were a single entity rather than a huge continent made up of incredibly varied and disparate peoples across terrain that runs the gamut from bone-dry desert to rainforest, and much in between. The received wisdom seems to be that there are pockets of progress and prosperity dotted across its fifty-odd countries, but that most Africans are yet to reap the benefits of their postcolonial freedoms and share in economic prosperity derived from the continent's enormous reserves of human and natural resources. Many countries are riven with civil war because colonial boundaries were drawn with little regard for local ethnic or tribal history, and the "strongman" in Africa developed an often-justifiable reputation for greed and corruption.

Every now and then the West does sit up and take notice of Africa and its problems—perhaps most famously as a result of reporting on the unfolding famine in Ethiopia in 1984, which led to the Band Aid, Live Aid, and USA for Africa charity initiatives, raising millions of dollars. Some twenty years later the conscience of the West was pricked again, this time by a growing humanitarian disaster in a province in the west of Sudan known as Darfur.

Sudan is enormous, covering a million square miles from its Red Sea coastline in the east to the vast desert wastes of the Sahara in the north and west of the country. Darfur itself, bordering Chad, Libya, and the Central African Republic, is the size of Spain. By the end of 2004 Sudan was emerging from a twenty-year civil war between the largely Islamist north, including the capital Khartoum, and the Christian south. Darfur was stuck between the two but not really included in the negotiations between the capital and the south, which would eventually lead to the creation of the new country of South Sudan in 2011.

Darfur wanted a share of the economic development that had been promised to the south, but the government in Khartoum resisted. In response the Sudan Liberation Movement (later Army, or SLA) emerged from several indigenous ethnic groups in Darfur and began attacking some of the garrisons run by the north, claiming the government was oppressing the country's non-Arab population. Khartoum retaliated and embarked upon a killing spree in Darfur and was subsequently accused of ethnic cleansing. The government began to train an Arabic militia, known as the Janjaweed, which has been translated as "devils on horses"—mounted armed raiders who were sent to attack and destroy villages suspected of harboring anti-government insurgents. They were given free rein to loot and kill and rape as much as they wanted. The Sudanese army sent in helicopter gunships to cause as much damage as they could and then the Janjaweed would ride into the ensuing chaos on horses and camels and execute any survivors.

As always happens, innocent people caught up in this carnage began to pack up whatever they could carry and move somewhere safer. The border between Chad and Sudan, on the western edge of Darfur, became a magnet for refugees. When I volunteered to go there with MSF in 2005, there were around two million people strung along the border with Chad and at least a million more who had already crossed into eastern Chad.

Our little hospital in Adré on the border with Sudan coped with thousands of patients all day, every day, in blistering heat. There was a surgical team with one surgeon, a nurse, an anesthesiologist, and some local staff. There was also a local doctor who dealt with all the diseases from the refugee camps, including significant malnutrition. Next door to our hut, which doubled as an operating room and recovery room, was the maternity suite. This had four midwives who worked around the clock. Most of the surgical work revolved around obstetrics—again I was reminded of how crucial it is to have a depth and breadth of knowledge of this vital area of medicine. To be able to safely perform a C-section and deal with the consequences of postpartum hemorrhage was a skill I had to call upon at all times of the day and night. But here the situation was truly terrible, much worse than it had been when I was in Afghanistan. We were asked to do maybe four or five Cesareans a day and, of those, we had a mortality rate of perhaps 25 percent. Malnutrition accompanied by malaria and sepsis associated with obstructed labor was the major cause of death.

We saw girls from as young as nine who had been raped by either Sudanese soldiers or the Janjaweed. Some fell pregnant, but their pelvises were not developed enough for natural, full-term births—the baby's head compared to the size of the pelvis was just too big, and would get stuck in the first stage of childbirth. These pregnant children would labor for hours and hours trying to deliver their babies. More often than not, the labor would continue for several days until they left their camp on a horse and cart to be brought down to our little hospital.

Sometimes the patient was so septic that the baby had died in utero before reaching us, and I would then have to do a fetal necrosectomy, an operation I thought had been consigned to the history books. It would begin with a vaginal examination which revealed not a healthy baby ready to begin its life but a stinking mass at the cervix: the unborn baby had already died and was becoming gangrenous. The operation involves making a hole through the fontanelle of the baby's skull using a large pair of scissors, which decompresses the head and allows the brain to be extruded. Clamps are then put around the cranium and the baby is pulled out. It is almost impossible to describe dispassionately and clearly how horrendous the experience is for the mother, and how deeply traumatic the operation is for the surgical staff who have to do it. It was a vision of surgical hell, and did not get any better for the eight weeks that I was there.

On top of this emotional torture, there was the physical assault of the climate. Our mission headquarters had been constructed with little regard for who might live in it. My bedroom was in a brick building with a shiny aluminum corrugated roof. The roof was supposed to reflect the sunlight but in fact turned the building into an oven, with the temperature averaging around 110 degrees, day and night. We used to stop operating between noon and three o'clock in the afternoon because the temperature in this period would go up to something like 130 degrees Fahrenheit.

I would come back having had a light meal and strip off completely and sit on a plastic chair with holes in it so the sweat just dripped off me onto the floor. There was no wind at all, and I was surrounded by bottles of water to replenish the liters of fluids I would sweat out through the chair. The nights were even worse, because the mosquito net kept in a lot of the heat and I would lie on a rubber mat and squish around in a puddle of sweat.

After one particularly heavy day, which had started early, I developed a headache so severe I could not continue to work. I told the anesthesiologist how I was feeling, and we decided to close the operating room for the night. I went to lie down but then had severe vomiting and intense muscle cramps in my arms and legs. I had a small amount to drink but vomited that back up instantly. Compounding my physical discomfort was my anger and irritability at the desperate state of the young women and girls we were trying so hard to treat and save from the horrific consequences of sexual violence.

By three in the morning I was hallucinating and seeing tractors with enormous wheels plowing through the mud in my room. It went on and on. As the sun rose at four and the donkeys started braying, I began to see elephants in my room. When I missed breakfast at eight, the head of mission came to find me on the verge of slipping into a coma. I was suffering from hyperthermia and dehydration, and if I hadn't been treated straightaway I would have gone into irreversible heatstroke and died. The anesthesiologist immediately took control and admitted me to my own ward, where I was catheterized and attached to an intravenous drip, pouring in the liters of saline that saved my life.

Soon after I recovered, I was asked to examine a girl aged about thirteen, who needed a Cesarean because she had been in labor for around three days. Although the cervix was fully dilated, the midwives could just feel the baby's head and thought that the baby was still alive. I approached this beautiful young girl, and made a motion to greet her by holding her hand, but she pulled away from me violently and, before I could explain who I was, spat in my face.

I was so shocked that I recoiled and promptly left the tent. It took me several minutes to recover. I remember going to find my anesthesiologist, who was from Lyon. He very gently tried to put it in context, saying that she probably hated all men, having undoubtedly been raped, and that her family were almost certainly all dead.

Still shaken, I needed a bit of a break before going back to examine her, so we went back to our mission headquarters a few hundred meters away. For half an hour or so we talked about the tragedy unfurling around us. I asked my anesthesiologist colleague to come back with me as the girl would need a spinal anesthesia before I could operate. But when we walked into the tent we saw that she now had a sheet drawn over her. I pulled it back and to my horror found that she had just died. My legs gave way and I slumped to the ground, holding on to the wheel of her gurney as I sobbed.

Very rarely do I cry on a mission, but the work in Chad was becoming almost too much to bear. My tears were a release after the weeks of emotional torture and stress that I had been subjecting myself to, which we were all going through. The week before this tragic episode, a woman had died on the operating table following a Cesarean. She had malaria, she was anemic, and I think this was her sixth or seventh child. It was her third Cesarean, and I was pushed into operating on her by the midwife. We had no ultrasound scanning machine; everything was done by physical examination. Four of her children were waiting outside the operating room. We had only one unit of blood available for her and there was no other blood in the blood bank.

She had had two Pfannenstiel incisions across the top of the pubis before, and so I elected to perform a midline incision as I felt it would be the safest option. It was all done under a spinal anesthesia, with the patient conscious throughout. All seemed to be going well until I made my incision into the lower segment of the uterus. As I've mentioned before, this lower segment usually has less muscle and bleeds less. There was a lot of scar tissue that I needed to go through first, however, and the bladder seemed to be stuck, so I carefully moved it aside. But once I had entered the uterus, I encountered considerable bleeding. Usually, the baby is sitting just underneath the incision, and gently separating it with your fingers allows good access into the uterus to find the head to deliver the baby. On this occasion, though, blood was pouring out. Because of the lack of staff, it was just me and the anesthesiologist and a table full of instruments in the room.

I pressed on the bleeding uterus with a big pack and told my colleague that I needed help now. We both shouted for assistance, but nobody came for at least ten minutes. The only person we could find was a young boy who worked as a cleaner. He had never scrubbed up before. The anesthesiologist supervised him as he washed his hands and helped him put on sterile surgical gloves and gown. I told him that I was going to place his hands where I wanted them and that he must not move them. I didn't even have a good suction device to help remove the blood, just a foot-activated device that I rapidly pumped to get some sort of suction going.

I couldn't understand why she was bleeding so much, but then it dawned on me. I had gone through the placenta, which must have been stuck to the scar from her previous C-sections. I was furious with myself; I should have thought about this.

With my new assistant's hand pressing on the incision I had already made to try and stop the bleeding, which was now a torrent, I made another incision in the top of her uterus to try to cut down through the muscle to find the baby. But things were now spinning out of control. A full-term uterus normally has a blood supply of around 600ml per minute. The patient had probably lost well over two liters of blood by this time. Panic set in, and I had an awful sinking feeling that this poor woman was going to die in front of me. The anesthesiologist quickly put her to sleep; he had no ventilator and was having to ventilate by hand, and there was no proper monitoring equipment.

Finally I located the baby and brought it out through a torrent of blood. I tried desperately to stop the bleeding with a running stitch into the uterus, and at one stage I thought I was winning the battle. The anesthesiologist administered the usual drugs to make the uterus contract, but it remained very floppy and the lower segment was still bleeding significantly. After only a few minutes he looked at me and shook his head. She had died, and the baby, too.

The rest of the operation was completed in silence. It had been an utter disaster. I sewed up her belly to make her look as normal as possible. How was I going to tell her children, who were still waiting outside? I was covered in blood from head to toe, so I quickly changed into clean scrubs and left the OR to explain what had happened. The oldest child was around ten. I asked where his father was, and the boy told me he had been killed by the Janjaweed.

Later that week I tried very hard to find out what had happened to the woman's children. I felt entirely responsible and wanted to give them money through the UNHCR, which was running the camps. I gave all the cash I had with me, about £300, to an official and said I was going to set up a bank draft when I got home to try to help them. As it was, when I did get home, I spent quite a lot of time trying to track them down, but they had been sucked back into the maw of the camps and simply disappeared.

Even years later I still have a feeling of despair when I think about this case. And I was not alone in being affected. After the abortive operation the anesthesiologist and I walked in stunned silence back to the mission headquarters. I could feel the tension coming off his body in waves as we approached several expat volunteers sitting at a table, drinking and smoking. As we reached them he completely lost it, overturning the table and sending ashtrays and beer flying into the air, screaming and yelling and smashing up chairs on the veranda and anything else he could get his hands on. I knew exactly how he felt.

This exceptionally difficult mission at last came to its end, and after I got back to London I went for a debriefing at the MSF headquarters. These are absolutely standard after every deployment, and usually last about forty-five minutes. I had had an outpatients' clinic beforehand so I arrived at their offices in a smart suit and tie.

I left the little room where the debriefing took place around six hours later in a completely disheveled state. I could not control myself. I bawled my eyes out for about four hours, and felt so sorry for the two MSF women who had to listen to me unburden myself of the stress, the horror, and the guilt.

I felt so wretched about my time in Adré, that—perhaps perversely—I decided I wanted to go back to Darfur the following year. I still don't know if this was about making amends or exorcizing demons—probably a bit of both. I ended up working in a small town called Zalingeii, which had become a point of refuge for many of the other villages that had been destroyed. By this point, the SLA had positioned themselves in a mountain range called the Jebel Marra. They had launched attacks from their hiding place in these mountains against the Sudanese army and the Janjaweed, and had been quite successful. They had, though, suffered significant casualties and requested help from MSF. We had to go to them because if the positions of the SLA soldiers were known and they were caught, they would have been killed.

The roads were so dangerous that we had to fly by helicopter to Zalingeii, and it was obvious from the air that whole villages had been burned to the ground in a scorched-earth policy. There's no doubt in my mind that this was a genocide of Arabic against black Africans in Darfur, for which the government of Sudan and the Janjaweed bear complete responsibility.

Zalingeii was a town of around 20,000 people and was therefore a little more secure. Villages of fewer than a thousand were very often leveled to the ground. Later in the mission, I happened to be visiting one such village when the Janjaweed arrived on horseback. There must have been at least thirty of them and they rode in like a cavalry charge with guns blazing. People were running for their lives, and we decided not to confront the militiamen but to take cover behind our vehicles. After what felt like hours but could not have been more than twenty minutes, some thirty-five villagers lay dead and around sixty were wounded.

The leader of the Janjaweed raid came up to the four of us cowering behind the vehicles and demanded to know who we were. One of our nurses started crying uncontrollably and I had that feeling of impending doom in the pit of my stomach. I had felt that sensation many times before and would do so many times again. My legs turned to jelly and started to shake. Being surrounded by wild-eyed, heavily armed men, who had just killed over a score of people in scorching temperatures of 100-plus degrees, was a terrifying experience. After explaining that we were humanitarians, there only to help people and with no political or religious agenda, we were allowed to move on. I looked behind me as we hurriedly left, and noticed the Janjaweed kneeling down in the sand to pray, no doubt in praise for their glorious victory.

As well as doing what we could in Zalingeii, there was also the option to work as a mobile surgical team in the areas where the SLA was operating. The project manager asked me if I would be up for it, because if I wasn't, we wouldn't be going. He couldn't guarantee our safety but had had assurances from the SLA that as soon as we reached the mountains we would be offered protection. There had been shelling recently from government troops, which of course could not be stopped. The project manager said he had also contacted the Sudanese (government) army—they had said they wouldn't target us directly but if we were in the area when the shelling started, they couldn't guarantee our safety either. The Sudanese had been told the date we'd be traveling, and that was it. It would be a hazardous trip.

I went back to my dungeon-like little room in the mission headquarters to sleep on it. What was I going to do? It was reasonably safe where we were, there was lots to do, and we were doing good work. Out on the road, helping the rebels, was an entirely different game, perhaps irresponsibly risky. But I knew what my decision would be as soon as I felt that little pressure-cooker of excitement building within me. It always happens when I get a sniff of a mission—I could not resist.

We spent the next day working out what equipment we were going to take with us, particularly the drugs we would need, including Ketamine and diazepam, and lots of local anesthesia. Ketamine, the so-called "horse tranquilizer," is the mainstay of anesthesia in this sort of work. It works on a dose-to-weight ratio and sedates the patient just enough to make it possible to do major surgery and it can be topped up depending on the length of the procedure. When used appropriately, it is a very safe drug. Diazepam, or Valium, is a short-acting sedative that initiates the sedation before Ketamine takes over. I packed as many surgical instruments and sutures as I thought I would need, and some sterile drapes and gowns. We picked up another MSF expat nurse who had agreed to come and act as our anesthesiologist, and so two nurses, a vehicle full of surgical equipment, and I left for the hills.

It was a long drive that took a couple of hours along a straight, dusty red road. We passed many burned-out villages before reaching SLA country and then began to climb a mountain track toward the rebel-held area. There was a checkpoint farther up the road, but we couldn't see who was manning it. As we got closer four children jumped out of a ditch next to it, carrying AK-47s. They did not look as callous as some of the children I'd seen in Liberia—those kids had been totally crazy. These boys looked about ten years old and had obviously not known that we were coming. They raised their weapons and pointed them at us as we approached.

What the hell do we do now? I wondered. Stop and slam the vehicle into reverse, like we had back in Sarajevo? Carry on as if we had every right to be there? Or put our foot down on the accelerator and blast our way through?

The driver spoke Arabic fluently but became very stressed. He stopped the car before we reached the checkpoint. We told him to carry on but he just froze. Perhaps they had heard we were coming, perhaps not. Children with weapons are probably the most dangerous of all—they have not always developed an understanding of right and wrong and will often blindly follow an order to the extreme.

It was a very tense moment; none of us knew exactly what to do. We edged forward until we got to the checkpoint. The driver spoke to one of the boys, who clearly didn't understand. There was a tree across the road that acted as a roadblock, but there was a small gap just big enough for our car to get through. We edged forward toward the gap and as soon as we were past it we screamed at the driver to floor it. We roared away in a cloud of dust—I don't know whether the boys fired at us or not, but soon we had rounded a bend and were safe.

We continued our journey until we came to another checkpoint, but this time it was manned by people who knew who we were and were expecting us. They took us on to a small village high in the mountains. For the first time, the temperature was pleasant, not unlike a nice summer's day back home.

We got to work. I had a fully armed SLA rebel as an escort, taking me to various small huts in the village, which had lots of men languishing in them, suffering mainly from gunshot wounds. Some had been there for days. I counted around twenty patients who needed surgery and tried to figure out where I was going to operate on them. The only thing I could see that might be used as an operating table was a concrete block about the size of a dining table, which was solid and stable enough to take a patient and the right sort of height. The problem was that it was outside, in full view of other members of the village.

For the next six hours or so I worked through the list of operations. Some patients had gangrene setting in and needed amputations; it was really the only way to get rid of the infection. They were all very cooperative and understood that this was probably their only chance of getting proper medical care. Our volunteer nurse anesthetist had never actually administered anesthesia before, but we followed strict protocols and she did a great job.

Before long, the concrete operating table became quite the spectacle. When we began there were perhaps a few people watching from a small hill nearby, but after a few hours we had an audience of hundreds. I just had to ignore what was going on around me and concentrate on the patient. We used a couple of locals to fan all the flies away, and after a while we had more fly-fanners than we could deal with. But by the end of the day nobody had died, and all the wounds were dressed and cleaned.

We came back a few days later and the patients lined up obediently to have their dressings changed. They gave us food and coffee and even gifts to show their gratitude. It was the first and last time I have operated al fresco. And it was one of the more peculiar experiences of my career to operate in the open with fully armed SLA soldiers with heavy machine guns strapped to their waists holding up a tarpaulin so that I could do my work in its shade. It was surreal, but oddly enjoyable, and I thought to myself, *This is what humanitarian work is all about.* Helping people who can't help themselves and taking a risk to do it.

As the mission neared its end I began to feel better about my time in Darfur: it had been so much more constructive than the previous year, over the border in Chad. Nonetheless, I was ready to go home. However, I discovered that, as sometimes happens, before flying out of Khartoum I was to have a few days of R&R provided by the aid agency. I was taken to a safe house in a small town called Nyala. It looked like a decrepit old colonial mansion, with many rooms. I was to be the only person there for the next three days. I felt exhausted and spent at least the first twenty-four hours in bed, with a big ceiling fan whirring above my head. There were some provisions left for me but that was about it. On a bookshelf of sun-bleached and dog-eared paperbacks, I found a copy of *The Stranger* by Albert Camus, a novel I found so utterly transfixing that the hours seemed to evaporate as I sat with it in my grasp.

I had developed a few stomach troubles, and spent a fair bit of time reading the book on the toilet. This was a pretty basic affair outside the main house in a concrete shed with a creaky wooden door. As in many places without running water it was basically a pit latrine, a cesspool of indeterminate depth and age, with a very old wooden seat with a hole in it perched on top of some brickwork. It was dark, with only a few slivers of light coming through the splintered wooden paneling to read by.

On one occasion when I was in there, I became aware of a noise very similar to that of a Wellington boot squelching through mud, coming from the dark below my bottom. I didn't give it too much thought, not really wanting to dwell on what was down there.

The next time I returned the noise beneath me was significantly louder. I walked back to the house and picked up a box of matches from the kitchen. I went back to the lavatory and with the door open lit a match to see what was going on.

The surface of the cesspool was much higher and closer than I had thought. I thought I saw something stir. I lit another match and peered in, holding my breath against the stench. My fight-or-flight reaction kicked in as soon as I registered what I was looking at, and I ran. For there, probably a foot away from where my backside would have been when sitting on the toilet, was the biggest python that I have ever seen, writhing in the filth below. Its body was at least two feet in circumference and its head was near the hole in the wooden seat. The consequences do not bear thinking about. But what a way to go!

I was back in Africa again in 2008, this time working in a small town called Rutshuru in North Kivu, a province of the Democratic Republic of the Congo that abuts Rwanda. Fourteen years earlier, in the genocidal slaughter of Tutsis by Hutus, nearly a million people had been killed during a hundred days of bloodshed. Tensions were still very high, and there was significant fighting from a rebel group led by Laurent Nkunda, a renegade warlord and ethnic Tutsi who liked to be called "The Chairman." He had accused the Congolese government of failing to protect the Tutsi people from Hutu militias that had escaped to the DRC after taking part in the genocide. His group was much better trained and equipped than the government troops, a motley bunch of defeated soldiers, rebels, and militias left over from back-to-back wars that had left millions dead. It was a disjointed, undisciplined, demoralized, and poorly paid outfit. By contrast it was believed that Nkunda, who had been implicated in numerous war crimes, had a group of highly trained and disciplined fighters who were receiving arms from Rwanda. It appeared that the Congolese army at the time and the Hutu rebels who controlled large parts of North Kivu were part of the same group.

There was intense fighting around the whole of the province, which predictably caused a mass exodus of people from their homes in eastern

Congo. When we were traveling up from Goma along a dirt track flanked by dense undergrowth, we could see the Congolese army dressed in green fatigues and green helmets at hundred-yard intervals. There were numerous checkpoints, too, and our driver, who was obviously well known locally, waved as we were let through all of them on our way to Rutshuru.

En route, we also saw occasional groups of people pushing all their wares on rickety wooden scooters called *chukudus*. The main frame is cut from eucalyptus with a machete, while the wheels are sculpted from a hardwood the locals call mamba. The wheels are wrapped in tread cut from old tires. The largest *chukudus* can carry as much as 1,700 pounds—they are a crucial form of transport in the eastern DRC, and indeed in 2009 President Joseph Kabila had a monument of a *chukuda* erected in the center of Goma, to symbolize the hard work of the people in the area. Now, though, they were not being used to carry charcoal, bananas, or other goods, they were being used as escape vehicles for families with all their belongings. The look on the people's faces said it all—they were scared, not only because of the continued fighting but also because they did not trust either side to protect them. There were stories of both sides killing and raping and stealing from civilians.

Although there was a general tension in the air, the hospital in Rutshuru turned out to be a rather peaceful and tranquil place, set in a beautiful part of the jungle with a mud road leading to a gate surrounded by high brick walls. In the briefing I was told that I would really enjoy this mission, as it had a steady throughput of patients. A Congolese surgeon was already there, and he turned out to be extremely good and technically very sound. He told me one evening that he had been there continuously for six months, and was desperate to see his family, who lived in the west of the country. I immediately replied that of course he must have a break. There was a junior expat surgeon with me and I was certain that the two of us would manage quite happily.

The team also comprised two nurses and a physical therapist who were living down the road, again in the most idyllic setting. My own hut was surrounded by palm trees and spectacular undergrowth, and I grew to love the walk of a hundred or so yards to the shower room, which had nothing but a cold water tap and a bucket. But we were in the tropics; it was exhilarating to fill up the bucket and wait for a moment before I summoned enough courage to throw the whole lot over my head and body.

Before the local surgeon left to see his family, I did some ward rounds with him so that he could hand over the patients to me. He was very worried about one of the young men, who'd had his arm bitten off by a hippopotamus several weeks before. He was lying in bed on the ward while his mother fed him *fufu*, a dough made with boiled cassava and flour, which was also to become our staple diet over the coming weeks. His mother told us that he had gone off his food in the last twenty-four hours and that she was very worried about him not eating.

After I had looked more closely, I began to fear that both mother and son were unaware of the gravity of his situation. The young man, who was about sixteen years old, had been operated on several times, each procedure taking off a bit more of his left arm. I asked the nurse to take the dressing off and had to take several steps back when the sickly-sweet smell of gangrene hit my nostrils.

He had about 10cm of his left arm remaining, but the skin was turning much darker than his normal skin tone and there was some blistering on the surface. The muscle was also black, a sign of decomposition. I could not see the bone of his humerus, which appeared to have been removed by previous surgeons.

I looked at the local surgeon. "I'm pretty sure he has gas gangrene," I said. "It won't be long until he dies."

"Yes," he replied, "but there's nothing more we can do."

We carried on the rest of our ward round, seeing patients my colleague had operated upon and also the patients of the volunteer who had preceded me. They were mainly orthopedic patients in traction for their fractured femurs or thigh bones. It was strange seeing as many as forty patients on a ward all in traction. It would never be like this in a Western hospital—the fractures would have been fixed internally with a metal rod and the patients probably discharged within a couple of days. These people were going to be here for two or three months before they could go home.

We then walked around the hospital's maternity unit, where the midwife showed us the next three patients, all of whom were in some distress. The partogram, a chart used by midwives to assess ongoing labor, indicates which patients are progressing and which are not. Two of the women required immediate Cesarean sections.

This was obviously not a mission for the novice. In such close-knit communities the word goes out very quickly if a surgeon causes problems or has difficulty in operating. There is no room for error. The local surgeon said he would do one of the Cesareans, as he knew the patient, and I could do the other. I asked whether I could assist him but he said he was fine, and suggested I carry on the ward round while the woman was prepped.

I went around the intensive care unit, which was unlike any ICU I had seen in the UK. There was one nurse for twenty beds. There were no ventilators, no banks of syringe drivers, no one-to-one nursing. It did, though, have charts that had been beautifully drawn by the single nurse, who measured all the patients' observations correctly, including pulse, blood pressure, temperature, and urine output, and all the fluid coming out of drains and nasogastric tubes. She wore a straw hat and a white coat and was clearly very experienced. She knew whether a patient was sick or not, and I began to understand how she managed such a workload.

After about half an hour I was told that my patient was ready for her Cesarean: she was on the operating table having her spinal anesthesia. The local surgeon hung around to watch me do it. I paused to gather myself; it was probably the first C-section I had done in two years—since my last trip to Africa, in fact.

I remember this operation well because it was difficult. The baby's head was firmly fixed down into the pelvis; the midwife told me that the mother had been fully dilated several hours before but all she could feel was the infant's scalp coming through the cervix. The head was stuck. I made a Pfannenstiel incision, found the lower segment of the uterus and cut into it. I put my left hand into the uterus to try to feel the baby's head. It was well and truly stuck, and I was unable to budge it.

My mind flashed back to that awful day in Darfur three years earlier, when my patient's postpartum bleeding had proved catastrophic. My heart began to beat very quickly as I realized I was up against the clock. I had to get this baby out. I looked around but the local surgeon had gone, so I spent another minute or so trying desperately to dislodge the head.

Then the nurse who was with me put his hand into the uterus as well, and lo and behold, the head of the baby popped free. The nurse smiled at me behind his mask and said, "*Vide*," which in French means vacuum. He had ingeniously slipped his fingers behind the baby's head, allowing some air to get between the head and the pelvis and break the seal. It's a trick I will never forget.

I met up with the local surgeon and, a little embarrassed, told him about the nurse and the vacuum trick. He didn't seem surprised and told me that if push came to shove, I could trust the nurse to do an operation. With that, he said he was going off to see his family and I wished him all the best.

I did a few more operations that day and then went back to my hut. But I couldn't stop thinking about that young man and his ruined arm. I knew that he only had a few days to live. The gangrene would induce septicemia, his kidneys would fail, and he would die, probably a slow and agonizing death. What he really needed was to have the whole of that upper arm removed, including the shoulder, an operation called a forequarter amputation. Despite all my training, I had missed out on how to do this procedure—and also how to do a hindquarter amputation, which is taking off a whole hip and leg. To compound this, I had also forgotten to bring the reference books that I usually carry around with me on a USB drive. Without the operation the boy would certainly die, but I did not know how to do it.

It suddenly came to me that I knew just the person to ask. My colleague Meirion Thomas was the professor of surgery at the Royal Marsden Hospital in London. He probably had more experience of doing this operation than anyone in the world. I had worked with Meirion for a long time; we knew each other very well and had operated together many times—it just happened to be the case that a forequarter amputation wasn't one of them.

I tried to call him several times but could not get through; each time I heard someone saying, in French, that it was not possible to connect. Time was passing for me, but it was running out for the boy. I was despairing by this point and decided to try a text from my Nokia phone. It was pouring rain outside and the noise of the rain on the roof of my hut was deafening as I typed "can you take me through a forequarter amputation using text." I sent the message at around six o'clock in the evening and went to bed at about eleven, after performing another C-section. At around midnight my phone, which hadn't made a sound for days, suddenly pinged. Amazingly, a text had arrived from Meirion. It read:

> Start on clavicle. Remove middle third. Control and divide subsc art and vein. Divide large nerve trunks around these as prox as poses. Then come onto chest wall immed anterior and divide Pec maj origin from remaining clav. Divide pec minor insertion and (very imp) divide origin and get deep to serrates anterior. Your hand sweeps behind scapula. Divide all muscles attached to scapula. Stop muscle bleeding with count suture. Easy! Good luck. Meirion

So there it was, instructions for how to do a forequarter amputation. What I didn't quite understand was where to make the actual cuts. I excitedly bounced out of bed, put the light on, and grabbed a newspaper that I had brought with me from the UK. I placed it on the floor and tried to summon up a picture of the patient and his arm. Now that I had the way to do it, I needed to determine how I was going to close the wound. I moved around my pieces of paper until I worked out where I should make the cut and where the flaps would be, so I could close the wound once I had removed the whole of his shoulder and scapula.

I went to bed excited but woke up the next morning feeling very apprehensive. It's all well and good doing the operation, but many of these patients require intensive postoperative monitoring and support, and they can lose a lot of blood and require massive transfusions. Would he make it through? Did we have enough blood?

I went for my usual bracing shower and waited for the car to take us to the hospital. My first visit was to my young patient, who was much worse than he had been the day before. It was now or never. I went to the operating room and found one of the two nurse anesthetists that worked with us. They were very experienced and I told them what I would like to do.

"We've never done anything so big before," came the answer, "and we don't have much blood." I took on board what they said. It was tricky. If I didn't perform the surgery, the boy would definitely die. On the other hand, if I did the surgery and the boy died as a result, and it emerged that the hospital had never attempted such a procedure before, it risked changing the whole relationship between me, the hospital, and the local community. In many ways it would have been much easier to have left the boy to die. But I knew I couldn't do that. I had to give him a chance of life.

I went to his mother and explained to her what I wanted to do, as well as the risks and the dilemmas. The anesthesiologist then came over and told me we had only one pint of blood available for the boy's blood group, and we couldn't get any more. He added that, though he was willing to help with the operation, we had to do it within the next hour or so because his wife was unwell and he needed to go home.

"But it will take at least three or four hours," I protested.

"All right," he said, "let's do it first thing in the morning."

I was unable to sleep that night for worrying about whether I was making the right decision. Back on the ward the next day I greeted the boy, who by this time was very septic. I was concerned that our opportunity to intervene had come and gone. Shall I, shan't I?

I walked outside to gather my thoughts, but by the time I came back in, the young man was already under general anesthesia. The decision had been made for me.

We didn't have the correct straps in the operating room and so had to use bedsheets to secure our patient in position, lying on his right side. I checked over all the instruments. My surgical nurse, in whom I now had a lot of confidence, was there to help. I had written out Meirion's text message on a piece of paper and stuck it on the operating wall so I could read it.

I began by making the incision over the clavicle and followed it transversely under the armpit and then around to above the scapula. I divided the clavicle with a Gigli saw, which is a grated metal wire attached to two handles which you pull rapidly backward and forward until it divides bones. I very carefully divided the subclavian artery and subclavian vein, making sure that I stopped the original stitch from coming off, which would have caused massive bleeding. I then divided all the nerve roots from the neck to the arm. Carefully following Meirion's instructions, I divided all the muscles necessary to remove the scapula and shoulder bones with the clavicle, taking with it what was by this time a completely infected arm and shoulder.

This part of the operation took about ninety minutes. I ended up holding this conglomeration of bone and tissue and infection and putting it in a bucket beside the patient. My nurse colleague was by this time pressing on all the bleeding points and, just as Meirion had said I should, I used a running suture to stop all the bleeding from the remaining muscle. There was a lot of blood on the floor and the anesthesiologist decided it was time to use the only pint we had.

I began to feel exhilarated as I realized that the skin flaps that I had created were in fact too big, and that closing the wound was going to be easy. In fact I had to remove some skin to get perfect wound closure. With two drains in position we slowly woke the patient up and kept him in the recovery room next door to the operating room for several hours. When he was completely awake, I went to tell his mother that all was well. Since he was only sixteen and didn't have any other major complications, such as the heart valve problems that can accompany such severe septicemia, he had a chance of making a full recovery. Indeed, by the time I left a few weeks later, he was up and about and looking extremely well and happy.

In the days that followed, however, our little hospital in Rutshuru went from being a tranquil place of healing to one overwhelmed with casualties. The fighting between the two groups of belligerents had taken a sharp upturn. Nkunda's group launched a significant offensive against the Congolese army and the Hutus fighting with them, and it wasn't long before we heard gunfire constantly. The gates of the hospital flew open and all sorts of wounded started piling through, some walking, some in cars or on the back of trucks. The hospital quickly became overstretched. Soon there were two or three people to a bed and many more on the floor. The fighting was by then continuous, to the point where we were not only treating the wounded but also harboring hundreds of civilians within the hospital compound. They came to escape the fighting and used the hospital as a sanctuary. Hundreds of families set themselves up with cooking pots and tarpaulin tents around the hospital grounds.

On one particular day we dealt with seventy-one individual gunshot wounds from fighting between the two groups, with the civilians caught in the middle, as ever. We had nowhere to put anyone and couldn't afford the luxury of trying to put soldiers from different sides into separate wards. Those who couldn't move because they were in traction had to stay in the same ward even if they were next to a man they might have been shooting at a few hours earlier, and mixed in among them were the civilians who'd been caught in the crossfire.

The Congolese army wore helmets but had no other protective body armor. It became a bit of a free-for-all, with gunshot wounds to arms, legs, heads, chest, and abdomen. They were typical of the sort of injuries caused by AK-47 bullets. If the bullet had not cut across a major blood vessel or the heart, then the patient had a good chance of survival, once they got to us. But we were seriously overstretched and the junior expat surgeon, who in normal circumstances would not have been allowed to operate on her own, had an operating room to herself. This work went on day in, day out, and throughout the night, as well as the C-section session that always occurred at around four o'clock in the morning.

In the middle of all this chaos, while I was operating, I felt a tap on the shoulder from the head of the mission with a message that my mother had become seriously ill. I left the surgery and called her sister in Carmarthen on the satellite phone. My aunt told me that Mum had fallen at home and had broken her hip and was also acutely unwell with a urinary problem.

My mother had not been well for around six or seven months. I had bought her a flat in London as she found Carmarthen very lonely after my father had died four years earlier. She became much more dependent on me. We would speak at least three times a day and we thought that staying near me would be good for her. But she found the flat, which overlooked the London helipad, far too noisy and was unwilling to go out much during the day because she became very nervous in such unfamiliar and crowded surroundings. She missed the smell of the country air and longed to see her sisters. So, back it was to Carmarthen.

She had been told that she had a urinary tract infection and went often to see her primary care physician, who prescribed antibiotics. I advised her to see a urologist in Carmarthen, but for some reason that appointment was never kept. She also had severe osteoporosis and had been on steroids for many years for rheumatoid arthritis, which left her hands deformed. When she was young my father and I would operate on her on the kitchen table, removing her rheumatoid nodules under local anesthesia. She had had both hips replaced while she was still in her thirties and was also suffering from arterial disease as one of the long-term effects of smoking.

My aunt told me that Mum had been admitted to Glangwili Hospital in Carmarthen, and that she was now very seriously ill and I should come home. Although I was exhausted, I immediately phoned MSF Paris to ask if they could arrange for me to leave straightaway, but was informed that it would take a week for my replacement to arrive. I phoned my aunt, who told me Mum would be dead within the week. What was I to do? There was no option, I had to go.

There was much discussion in the hospital office on the day I was due to leave. One debate concerned whether the road out was too dangerous; the other was about whether it was right to leave the hospital short-staffed. I tried to control myself, feeling that nothing was going to stop me leaving even if I had to walk home. I probably laid it on a bit thick but eventually they relented and a Land Cruiser was organized to take me down the perilous road from Rutshuru to Goma, where I would fly out the following day. The young expat surgeon would be in charge until my replacement arrived.

When the Land Cruiser pulled up, I noticed that the driver looked scared. We filled the back of the car with patients to take to Goma, too. One was a Congolese colonel who had been shot in the leg. I had repaired his artery and put him in a slab of plaster of Paris for the transfer as he also had a leg fracture. There was a woman who needed reconstructive surgery for a gunshot wound to her face, and a child with severe burns who needed careful management.

The five of us set off. The forty-five-mile journey was supposed to take around three hours, but in that time we covered only around ten miles. The road was absolutely packed with civilians trying to escape the violence. The driver jostled the vehicle between them as we tentatively made our way down the dirt track, trying to avoid children at the same time as trying to stay out of the deep puddles and rutted mud that would have ended our journey prematurely if we had gotten stuck. I felt myself getting very, very tired, and although we were being bounced around on the road, which seemed endless with its bright red mud, I actually fell asleep.

Before long I became aware that the car was going much faster, and when I opened my eyes there was a clear road ahead. Again I was amazed at the beauty of the country, its beautiful hills packed with dense green foliage. Mysteriously, the road was now eerily quiet, with not a person or vehicle to be seen. I was about to ask the driver where everyone had gone when we turned a corner and found a huge chain strung across the road.

Roadblocks are well known to aid workers and do not generally cause major issues; they are part of getting from A to B in a conflict zone. However, as we slowly approached, we realized that this did not look like a regular roadblock. Suddenly a man jumped out from the side of the road, near the tree that the chain was wrapped around. He looked totally crazy, with wide staring eyes, and he was carrying an AK-47 with belts of bullets around his shoulders and waist. I was always told you must never look into the eyes of anybody who is threatening you: never make eye contact because once you do, they have you.

I'm not sure if it was accidental or subconscious, but I could not stop myself from meeting the man's eye as he came toward us. I looked down and then back up, again transfixed by his eyes as he approached, his gun pointing directly at us. I was trying desperately to wind up the window but I was too late. He was talking in a language I did not understand and started shouting and screaming at me, the only non-African in the car. I could smell the strong whiff of booze on his breath and could feel his spittle on my cheek. He was ranting, in full flow, deranged. The gun barrel came through the open window and pressed against my neck.

In the Hollywood movie version of this scene I would have pulled some slick move, grabbing the barrel of the gun before jumping out of the car and decking this guy. But I realized there was nothing I could do. He had the weapon, he had his finger on the trigger, he could end my life within a fraction of a second. The muzzle pressed on my neck. I could feel my heart racing and my carotid arteries were pulsating so much that my head started bobbing backward and forward. I was sure that at any moment my life would end. I was completely catatonic, unable to move.

The wounded colonel in the back of the Land Cruiser started shouting at the man, who it seemed was a member of the Congolese army. Immediately, he lifted the gun from my neck and started waving it around inside the vehicle, at which point the driver flung open his door and sprinted off up the road. The colonel kept shouting and shouting—there was a lot of back-and-forth between the two of them as the man circled the car, still brandishing his gun. He checked inside but didn't open any bags. He looked at the child, who was now terrified as well as obviously badly burned, and the woman whose face was wrapped in bandages, and slowly everything seemed to calm down.

The colonel told me to drive, and so I shimmied into the driver's seat. I was so stressed and shaking so much that I could not start the engine. I became mute and was utterly incapable of following any basic instructions coming from the backseat. Finally I saw a start button. I pressed it and the engine growled into life. I put the car into first gear and the man with the gun dropped the chain to the ground. I slowly, slowly drove over the chain and continued driving, expecting a volley of shots any second. Around the next bend was our driver, peering out of the undergrowth. I felt tempted to drive straight past.

The rest of the journey was uneventful. Without a doubt I owe my life to the colonel, who I suppose was repaying me for saving his.

I finally made it back to Wales, and was so grateful to be able to see my mother before she died, which she did just two days later, on October 17,

2008. But I could not shake off a sense of guilt. While I had been making plans to go to the Congo, she had kept telling me about her urinary infection and that there were "bits" in her urine. But I did not put two and two together until I got the call about her being in the hospital and worked out that she must have developed a connection between her bladder and her colon, a so-called colovesical fistula. It usually occurs because of an inflammation of the colon called diverticular disease, which can eventually perforate into the bladder. It is incredible to me now, looking back on it, that I missed such an obvious and straightforward diagnosis, and I don't think I will ever get over not seeing it for what it was.

I was fifty-two years old when my mother died. I wasn't in a relationship, my flat was a place to sleep in rather than a home, and I felt unmoored. It's inevitable that the death of a parent makes you think about what you're doing and where you're going, what it's all for. I knew I was helping people both in the UK and abroad, and that work was immensely rewarding. But although I now had a lot of knowledge and experience, I could only be in one place at any given time.

How many more lives did I have? I couldn't keep cheating death forever.

I kept coming back to the nurse in the Congo with his vacuum-popping trick, and Meirion Thomas's text message. It wasn't enough just to go somewhere and help for a few weeks or months; it would only have lasting meaning if the local doctors I worked with could share in my knowledge and expertise, and the knowledge and expertise of all the other medical volunteers.

Back in 2002 I had run a course with the Red Cross to train British surgeons who were volunteering in the developing world and conflict zones. It would be even better, I now realized, to teach those who were on the front lines all the time.

-7-
TRAUMA SCHOOL

As usual, it began with a phone call. I was sitting at home watching the latest bit of fallout from the Arab Spring of 2011. The wave of protests had rippled out from its crucible in Tunisia and had spread eastward to Libya, where Colonel Muammar Gaddafi had been in power since 1969. As in Tunisia and Egypt, the cry went up: "The people want the fall of the regime!" They wanted freedom of expression, and the right to choose their own leader democratically. Protests in Benghazi, on the Mediterranean coast, had escalated since February, and by April the country was sliding toward a full-scale civil war.

Unusually, the call came directly from the MSF headquarters in Paris, rather than their London office. Was I available to go to Misrata, a port city of about 800,000 people that lies between Benghazi and Tripoli? I'd be going with an experienced surgical team, probably for a month, and within the next forty-eight hours.

I was told to rendezvous with the rest of the team in Valletta, Malta, from where we'd go on to Misrata by boat. I was delighted to hear that the British anesthesiologist Rachel Craven was coming, too. I had worked with Rachel several times over the years, and knew that her knowledge, skill, common sense, and calmness would be a great tonic in the days ahead.

Heathrow Airport was full of tourists and vacationers, and I felt the incongruity of knowing that our party was bound not for sun-loungers and cocktails but a war zone. Rachel and I were not sitting next to each other but our eyes met and a knowing look passed between us as we watched a fight break out between two passengers. The one in front was reclining his seat so the other could not fold down his tray table to eat his food properly. The passenger behind began pushing the offending seat backward and forward in a frenzied fashion until a flight attendant came to calm the situation. Usually it's when you come back from a war zone at the end of a mission that you are struck by the banality of life, and how ridiculous petty and pointless disputes like this seem.

Once we had arrived in Valletta, we were introduced to the rest of the team. There was an American surgeon and his wife, a retired professor of anesthesiology from Washington, an emergency physician, nurses, and a logistician. The following morning we were briefed on the situation on the ground in Misrata, which was changing by the minute. There was intense fighting in the streets, and significant casualties, chiefly from Gaddafi's tanks, which were rolling in. They also surrounded the city itself, firing heavy artillery on homes and other buildings. The rebels blocked the roads into the areas they held with trucks filled with sand to stop the tanks' advance, and there were regular firefights between the rebels and government troops.

The briefing officer told us we would leave Valletta for Misrata under the cover of darkness. The journey would take around twenty hours, and the crossing might be rough, so we should be prepared for some seasickness. Once there, a field officer would take us to a safe house.

Later that evening, we were taken down to the quayside to begin our journey aboard a fishing boat chartered by MSF, its flag indicating that it was a humanitarian vessel. The MSF logo was emblazoned on the front and back of the small bridge, where the captain was sitting. He'd agreed to take us in return for €300,000 cash.

We waited for dusk and watched the ropes being removed from the mooring on the side of the jetty. We all felt both excited and wary—we would be going directly into a war zone via one of the only routes in or out of the country, which was undoubtedly being watched by Gaddafi's troops. Before the boat sailed, we were all asked if any of us wanted to pull out—it was the point of no return. Despite feelings of intense trepidation no one did so, and the boat very slowly began to chug out of the harbor into the choppier waters of the open sea.

The captain's mate served dinner almost immediately, and we sat around the table downing boiled rice and chicken and drinking orangeade. After an hour or so, however, the sea became much more than choppy: we soon started to roll on the waves at an angle of around forty-five degrees, back and forth, back and forth. The waves grew higher and higher and all of us simultaneously began to get terribly seasick and bolted for the side of the boat. I asked the captain how many more hours there were to go, and he laughed and said, "Sixteen!"

I ventured on deck as dawn rose and was surprised to see a Royal Navy frigate on one side and a French warship on the other, escorting our tiny fishing boat. They would soon be leaving us, though, the captain told me, as we were about fifty nautical miles from Misrata harbor, which was a no-go area for NATO vessels. Sure enough, both ships soon veered off and we were on our own.

The sky was blue and the sea looked deep and dark as we sailed toward land. The captain and his mate kept a careful eye on the horizon through their binoculars, but then they started surreptitiously whispering to one another. I was given the binoculars so I could look for myself. Slowly, the outline of the city came into view. Smoke was billowing high into the sky, both from within the city and from around the harbor, where an oil refinery had been hit. It continued to burn for days after our arrival.

The closer we got, the more tense the captain and his first mate became. Our speed slowed from around fifteen knots to five, and then down to two as we approached the harbor entrance. As Rachel and I stood next to the captain looking at each other in an eyebrows-raised kind of way, she suddenly asked, "Do you think we've overdone it this time?" I wanted to say something to lighten the tone but found I couldn't. My heart was in my mouth.

(I did not discover the reason for the captain's anxiety until long after the mission, when Rachel phoned me at home: "Did you know that the entrance to Misrata harbor was mined?" she asked. NATO had apparently cleared them about two weeks after we left. How our little boat got through unscathed, I will never know.)

When we approached our mooring point on one side of the rectangular harbor, it seemed unusually quiet. Then I spotted a truck with a .50-caliber machine gun on the back being driven along the road on the opposite side, matching our speed as we came to dock. It was daubed in mud, to camouflage and hide any insignia. As the boat drew up against the quay, so did the truck. Suddenly, a group of cars and a truck arrived from nowhere. None of us knew what to expect next and we all held our breath. Then, a man wearing an MSF jacket emerged from one of the cars.

"Hello!" he shouted. "I am Mohammed, the field coordinator. Welcome to Misrata!"

Relieved, we left Mohammed's men to load the truck and sped off in the other cars to the MSF safe house in a residential area of the city. It was a fairly large building and was afforded some protection from shelling by neighboring houses. There was a kitchen, a sitting room, and several other rooms that were used as bedrooms. The majority of us men slept on mattresses on the floor of one room, sharing a very small bathroom. The women were in another room with, I noticed, rather better facilities.

After settling in we trooped down to the sitting room for a briefing. Mohammed told us that we were the first team that MSF had put into Misrata—indeed, the first into Libya since the war had started. To begin with, it was slightly unclear what our duties would be. There were two functioning hospitals in the city, Al-Hikma and Al-Abbad, both a few miles from the front line. Al-Hikma was a private hospital that had been taken over by the rebels and converted to a trauma unit, while Al-Abbad was a cancer hospital that had also been repurposed. It was up to us to work out where our surgical team would be most useful.

Mohammed also tried to bring us up-to-date on the security situation, but it wasn't long before we were all crouched down on the floor as tank shell after tank shell flew over the top of the house, some obviously quite high, but others worryingly close to roof level. The barrage went on for about thirty minutes and was a very eloquent substitute for a more formal briefing. Eventually, Mohammed was able to explain that we were lucky to get in that day, as there had been significant shelling of the port—only a couple of days earlier around twenty people had been killed and more wounded while waiting for a boat to take them to safety.

Mohammed explained that the rebels were not really soldiers at all; few of them had any training and they had hardly any proper weapons. They were ordinary hardworking people—carpenters, shopkeepers, mechanics, and waiters—who had never previously picked up a gun in their lives. Most of their arms came from dead pro-government troops. They had no military understanding of the situation and so were suffering many casualties, which was why we were there.

Despite their inexperience, however, Mohammed mentioned that the conflict was not as one-sided as one might think. What the rebels were lacking in equipment and military knowledge was made up for in their desire to overthrow Gaddafi, and they were willing to fight to the death.

The fighting in Misrata was at very close quarters, almost house-to-house, and, as the city was completely surrounded, the rebels had no way out. There was no place to go, apart from the sea, and this would be no Dunkirk. Gaddafi's forces were determined to annihilate the rebels, and automatically regarded anyone trying to carry on as normal and adopt a neutral position as anti-government and therefore a terrorist.

After a somewhat spartan meal of beans, biscuits, and black coffee, we went to our rooms. The first night in a war zone is for me always filled with a mixture of anxiety and exhilaration. I am only too aware that not only am I somewhere totally alien, but also witnessing history in the making; feelings of personal safety take second place.

The next day we went to the Al-Hikma Hospital. Mohammed took me to meet its director to discuss how the team could best be put to use. It wasn't the easiest of meetings, and got off to a disturbing start. The director looked at me and said "English? English?" and when I nodded he beckoned me to follow him. We went along to what turned out to be the hospital's morgue, adjacent to one of the meeting rooms. What we saw when he opened the door was appalling. It was full of dead bodies all piled on top of one another. I had never seen anything so horrific. I'm not sure whether he wanted to shock me or whether he was trying to convey just how dangerous this place was.

We were then shown around the rest of the hospital. I discovered there were two other expat agency teams already there, and I wondered how well we would all work together. Sometimes it can be quite difficult when other surgical teams are already in place who have developed their own ideas and practices. And at Al-Hikma, as is often the case in war zones, many of the senior local surgeons had already left, fearing for their families and having the resources to get out. As I would discover again in Syria, it's the junior staff who stay behind, and the ones here did not have much experience in trauma surgery. Before the war, Libya had been relatively peaceful, and they would have seen some blunt-force injuries from car crashes or the like, but nothing like the wounds we would now be dealing with.

The wards were full to capacity. We went to the intensive care unit, where, upon learning that I was a vascular surgeon, one of the doctors asked me my opinion on a man who had been shot through his left knee. The patient had already been operated on, and he had an external fixator in position from above to below the knee. The surgeon had apparently performed a graft to bypass the injured artery and vein. The man's left foot was white and cool compared with the other leg; his calf was very swollen and he was in considerable pain. The injury had happened the day before and he had been in one of the operating rooms for about eight hours through the night.

When I go to a war zone there's a certain amount of my own equipment that I take with me. I take my own surgical scrubs and a gas mask, and I take my loupes, which are lenses with four-times magnification that help me perform intricate surgery on small blood vessels and flaps used in plastic surgery. I take a light source, a kind of headlamp, so that I can continue to operate when the generators go down or the lights go off, and which also allows me to see deep into the crevices of a wound; and I take my Doppler machine, which allows me to hear the blood flow of the small distal vessels when the arteries do not have enough pressure to give a pulse. I carry it all around in a big, battered, old gray suitcase.

I now took out my Doppler machine to listen to the man's distal vessels. There was no blood flow into the foot at all that I could detect. I also noticed that no fasciotomy had been performed. Fasciotomies are crucial in cases of vascular trauma. The muscles in the leg are surrounded by a tight constrictive covering, or fascia. The fascia is a bit like hard plastic sheeting. If an arm or a leg or indeed any tissue has its blood supply cut off for an extended period, then the cells and muscles stop functioning normally and begin to swell up. The treatment for this is a fasciotomy, the division of the strong tissue surrounding the muscle in the leg. It's a relatively simple operation but needs to be done well. Without it, patients like the man with the gunshot wound in his knee will undoubtedly lose their leg.

Having examined the patient, I advised the ICU doctor that although it might already be too late, it was essential to perform a fasciotomy if we were to have any hope of avoiding amputation. I also asked which surgeon had been treating the man thus far. He shrugged and replied, "This is a war. It doesn't matter who did it or where he is now, the most important thing is to help the patient." Of course he was quite right, but having come across extremely alpha-male surgeons both at home and in the field, I felt it was only right that I should ask.

In a matter of minutes, the patient was being wheeled down to surgery while I found Mike, the American surgeon, and told him what I was about to do. He agreed that we should go ahead with the procedure and said that he would assist me. As we were scrubbing up, we suddenly became aware of a man shouting angrily in Arabic. Mike continued to scrub but I stopped and turned to confront the objector. It was the original surgeon on the case, who was furious. An Egyptian doctor in his mid-thirties, he demanded to know who I was. A British consultant vascular surgeon working for MSF, part of a team that had arrived that day, I replied. He was adamant that I had no right to operate on his patient and asked me to leave the OR. It was horribly tense.

Situations like this require considerable diplomacy. No matter how appalled you might be by a colleague's obvious mishandling of a case, you have to remain calm and courteous. Knowing that the patient's life was at risk, I was angry and concerned—my heart was beating faster and I could feel the hairs on my arms rising. But I had been here before and knew that the best option was to try to smile my way out.

"Before I leave your operating room," I said, "please would you show me how you will manage this patient's white foot, because I'd be very interested in learning your technique?"

He looked at the foot, unable to deny that there was a problem with the circulation, and shouted at the nurse to take the dressings off. He was going to expose the blood vessels to show us that the vein graft he had performed was working. Once he had done so, he turned to me triumphantly, inviting me to look. The blood vessels around the knee were indeed working well. However, he had left the artery exposed. It was bound to get infected, which meant that the join between the artery and vein graft would break down. The patient would probably bleed out from the secondary hemorrhage.

"Why is the foot still white?" I asked.

"It will get better," was the best he could come up with.

I then broached the idea of a fasciotomy because the leg was so swollen. I will never forget his reaction—he went red in the face and screamed "I never do fasciotomies!"

I considered replying, "Well, you do now," and punching him in the face, but I had to put the patient's interests first. I managed to restrict myself to glaring at him, while wondering how far I should push this. I squared my shoulders and said firmly, but calmly, "I'm very sorry, but I am a consultant surgeon with many more years' experience than you. In my opinion a fasciotomy is required and that is what I am going to do."

And with that I asked for the scalpel and made two long incisions on either side of the leg, cutting through the subcutaneous tissue until I reached the fascia and performed the fasciotomy. Alas, some of the muscle was already dead, and I showed my intemperate colleague, suggesting that they should now consider an above-knee amputation after speaking to the patient when he woke up. We finished the operation in complete silence and once I had dressed the wounds the surgeon walked out and I never saw him again.

The fasciotomy debacle was a foretaste of the MSF team's experience at Al-Hikma. I spent the rest of that first day walking around to see what was going on in the operating rooms and in the triage tent that had been set up in front of the hospital. The triage tent was full of equipment including ultrasound and portable X-ray machines. There were plenty of gurneys available for casualties. It looked professional, ready for action, and it wasn't long before we saw some.

We heard the sound of approaching ambulances, their sirens wailing in the distance. All of a sudden, the tent was a hive of activity with dozens of people arriving in anticipation of a mass-casualty event. There were clinicians wearing the logo of the International Medical Corps flocking around the entrance, others wearing the red shirts of the Italian humanitarian NGO EMERGENCY, and many Libyan medical students manning the gurneys.

Mike and I stood with the milling crowd as the ambulances rushed into the hospital. Some of them had cracked windshields, others looked significantly worse, with their radiators exposed where the front of the ambulance had been blown off by artillery fire. The whole place was soon in utter chaos; a crowd of over two hundred were at the front of the tent. There were people carrying AK-47s and other assault rifles, and more ambulances driving through the throng, which was scattering left and right. The noise was incredible, with voices shouting and screaming and sirens blaring. I held Mike's arm and suggested that, as we did not know anybody here, we should just watch and see how they coped.

It was obvious that most of the incoming casualties had been shot. I saw a man with a gunshot wound to the abdomen, who appeared to be conscious when he arrived but was soon surrounded by so many people it was difficult to see what was going on. A second man was wheeled in with what looked like a gunshot wound to his chest. He was unconscious and very pale, and I thought he might already be dead. But, again, he was quickly surrounded by so many people it was difficult to tell.

The triage tent began to fill up with other casualties. I pushed my way in to see how they were coping with the abdominal injury, and by the time I got there saw two surgeons making a very small incision just above the belly button. There was blood pouring out of the abdomen and being replaced with what looked like saline fluid. There was a tube attached to a suction machine that was not doing anything at all. I watched as the patient died on the gurney, unable to get closer because of the rows of people in front of me. The surgeons then moved on to the man who was shot in the chest and proceeded to try a thoracotomy. I had already concluded he was dead, but one of the surgeons—I'm not sure if he was a local surgeon or working for an NGO—made an incision to open the chest. It was far too low and the colon and stomach prolapsed out of the wound as external cardiac massage was tried. But there was no bleeding as the heart had stopped beating many minutes before.

Another man also had a gunshot wound to the chest. He was bleeding and in shock, but conscious and talking. One of the rules in resuscitation is that if a patient is conscious and can speak, then he has enough arterial pressure to supply the brain, even though he may have a low blood pressure from hemorrhage. This patient was talking and had a pressure dressing placed on the upper left part of the chest, near his shoulder. The majority of penetrating wounds to the chest can be managed with a chest drain. What comes out of the chest drain determines whether or not the patient needs his chest opened to stem the bleeding surgically. The majority of chest-wound bleeds will eventually stop on their own; mostly, they are the result of venous oozing from either fractured ribs or the lungs. Very rarely does one have an arterial source requiring stitches, and if it does, it's usually an intercostal artery below a fractured rib. Those patients who have penetrating injuries to the main blood vessels that leave the heart, such as the aorta, do not usually survive long enough to make it to hospital.

It was clear to me that the initial management of the wound should have been to use a chest drain. For some reason, though, one of the surgeons indicated that he wanted to take the patient to the operating room. Again, Mike and I decided not to say anything but to go with them into surgery to see what would happen next.

In trauma surgery, the usual body position is the shape of a crucifix with arms extended at right angles to the torso. This allows the surgeon to access both sides of the chest, the abdomen and pelvis, the arms and legs, head and neck. Very rarely are patients put on their side. On the way to the operating room I stopped for a short while and entered another room where a different NGO surgeon was working. His patient was having an exploratory operation to assess the damage caused from a gunshot wound to the abdomen. He seemed to be doing all right and I asked him about the patient's injuries. He told me most likely kidney and small bowel, as there was a large swelling in the flank and he was about to move the small bowel over so that he could see exactly where it was coming from. I asked him if I could help and he said no, because he had done this operation many times before. I left him to get on with it and caught up with the patient with the chest wound.

I was becoming increasingly unhappy with what I was seeing. The man had been laid on his side and a very large incision made on the left side of his chest. But there was very little bleeding in there; the surgeon went in and scooped out only around half a liter of clotted blood. Mike's wife was the scrub nurse for the procedure and we all watched, horrified, as an operation that should have taken five minutes to put in a chest drain took three hours of valuable surgery time in a hospital full of casualties.

I left the OR and walked back out into the fresh air, but before leaving the building I passed the operating room where I'd seen the man having the abdominal procedure. He was lying on the table, lifeless. I could only assume that the bullet had traversed a major artery or vein and that the patient had bled to death. The surgeon I'd spoken to was nowhere to be seen.

Later I saw an orthopedic surgeon, again from outside Libya, treating a femoral fracture caused by a high-velocity gunshot wound by inserting a rod down the middle of the femur. This is absolutely standard procedure, provided the environment is scrupulously clean, as it would be in any hospital in the UK. We have laminar flow operating rooms, which provide high air pressure inside the OR with vents to the outside that remove any bacteria. Orthopedic surgeons also wear a getup that resembles a spacesuit to keep everything absolutely sterile. Any bacteria in a metal prosthesis passed into the bone can cause osteomyelitis, a severe infection. An infected bone will not heal and the prosthesis will have to be removed, which is a disaster. Not only that, there is a high mortality risk. In trauma surgery in austere environments and war zones, where the whole place is dirty and only very basic equipment is used, it is a rule never to fit internal fixation rods.

This was trauma surgery, but it was trauma surgery performed by non-trauma surgeons. It was clear to me that they were making the wrong decisions, doing the wrong operations, and totally misunderstood the nature of war surgery. Concerned, I went to see the hospital manager to share my frustration at what I had seen. Unfortunately he gave me fairly short shrift, saying that all the international volunteers were trying their best and he was grateful for their help. I don't think he understood what I was talking about.

"I understand your point of view," I said, "but I'm sure we can achieve a significant improvement in survival rates if you give me the chance to try and talk to some of the surgeons."

But I couldn't get through to him—he simply said there was no space at Al-Hikma to do that, but I should go and try another hospital nearby.

We all left the hospital that evening feeling pretty despondent. It was dark by then and we almost got caught in the nightly curfew, but luckily managed to get through to the safe house. Once we got there, we immediately discussed our concerns with Mohammed, who agreed to ask the chief of surgery at Al-Abbad Hospital whether our team could go there. Fortunately, the answer was yes.

It was now very clear to me that in order to make a real difference in Libya—indeed, in any hostile environment—I had to do more than just operate on whoever happened to be put in front of me. That would help one person, but the much bigger goal was in trying to improve the whole system. Too many volunteers with good intentions were being put in situations outside their normal experience and were making poor decisions as a result. I had to try to change the whole modus operandi of the surgeons there. But how?

Apart from my own personal experience, having by this point been volunteering for nearly twenty years, I had another ace up my sleeve. I was the director of a course run by the Royal College of Surgeons in London called the Definitive Surgical Trauma Skills (DSTS) course. This course is mainly aimed at first-world surgeons, who will be dealing with victims of trauma, either blunt or penetrating. It teaches surgeons to evaluate difficult clinical scenarios and gives them the confidence to perform the correct operation. The course in the UK runs three or sometimes four times per year. It is a two-day course which teaches surgeons—from middle-grade registrars up to senior consultants—how to manage a patient with severe blood loss (half to three-quarters of their blood volume). There are scenarios around each individual trauma situation and surgeons then operate on fresh frozen cadavers using the techniques we teach them. Luckily, I had the DSTS course on a USB drive that I had brought with me. It would be a good place to start with the doctors at Al-Abbad and Al-Hikma.

Given that I'd already encountered some resistance to doing things differently, I knew it would be an uphill struggle. But I had to try. I contacted the director of Al-Hikma and told him that every day from midday onward I would be running a trauma training course at Al-Abbad, which his staff and his overseas volunteers would be welcome to attend. And I added that I'd also be happy to discuss their cases, if they wanted.

The next day, I found the lecture room at Al-Abbad and set up my laptop. I went through my notes and got ready to face my audience. Of course, nobody came. In fact, nobody came for the next three days. But on the fourth day, a few medical students turned up, and I was delighted to talk them through the course. And word then got around—there were actually useful things to be learned from the strange Brit with the laptop. Within three weeks the lecture room was full, with surgeons and students from both Al-Abbad and Al-Hikma.

The shift in mood was palpable. The general management of cases began to improve and it was very gratifying to see the local surgeons putting their newfound knowledge into practice—and its immediate effect. This was the future, I believed—not just parachuting into a war zone, saving the odd life, and then going home; it was about providing a legacy, leaving my temporary colleagues better equipped to deal with an ongoing situation that they themselves could not walk away from.

Before Libya, I don't think I would have had the confidence to try to effect such change. But I had a lot of missions under my belt, and the directorship of the DSTS course also gave me a boost: it helped silence that doubting inner voice that said, *Who are you to tell them what to do?* I had learned the importance of trying to take people with you and displaying tact and humility wherever possible. Wading in and barking orders helps no one; you have to build relationships, and trust, before anyone will become open to accepting that there might be a better way of doing things.

We were nearing the end of our mission. A few days before we were due to leave, we heard that Gaddafi's forces, which had by this point completely surrounded Misrata, were planning to shell the city and destroy it. That night we had an emergency meeting with Mohammed. There was still no way out of the city except via the port, but there was no way that a boat was going to come in and collect us, given the security situation. It was simply too dangerous. If worse came to worst, Mohammed told us, the French military would send in a helicopter to pick up the MSF team. We were a little skeptical about this, but it was our only hope, and we all prayed for our safety at lights out while listening to the constant *thud thud thud* of incoming artillery fire.

Fortunately NATO then swung into action, bombarding the Libyan government's tank positions for the next forty-eight hours. Every time the tanks fired an artillery shell, NATO responded with a precision strike on the source. The intelligence reports had suggested that the Tuesday before we were due to leave would see the big offensive, but it was probably the quietest day we had witnessed since we'd been there.

We continued working until Friday, our planned departure date. By that time the safe house was full of new expats arriving from all over the world. One of the new anesthesiologists was from Seattle. He had had a long journey, flying to Paris and then, like the rest of us, on to Malta, followed by the twenty-hour, very rough sea crossing. He took the mattress next to mine in the room we all shared. He seemed nice enough, but he sat up for half the night tapping away at his laptop, which seemed a bit strange. The screen glow lit up the room, too, which slightly unnerved us. There were very strict guidelines about lights out during the curfew. No one said anything, though. We were all so tired that we really didn't care by this point, and were in any case about to go home.

The following night—our last in Misrata—the new incoming project manager called a general meeting. This was very unusual; it had never happened on any previous mission and I wondered what it was all about. At 11:00 p.m. we all gathered in one of the house's larger rooms. There were about thirty of us, and each of us was asked in turn if we had done anything to jeopardize the security of the mission.

It was a strange question, and a difficult one to answer. We all felt that perhaps we *had* done something—taken a photograph or whatever—that maybe we shouldn't have. But to put the whole mission in jeopardy?

Rachel and I were sitting next to each other and gave each other an uncomfortable look as the question came around to us. "No," she said quickly, followed by me. "No, nothing." Almost all of us answered "No" until we came to the anesthesiologist from Seattle, who looked acutely uncomfortable.

"I may have done . . ." he said. "I was writing a blog about what was happening to us here in Misrata."

"But you've only been here for twelve hours," came the response. "Your blog was intercepted by NATO and alarm bells went off at the MSF headquarters. In your blog you mentioned who was here, where they were from, what roles they had, and so on. Do you not think that is a security lapse?"

It was an extremely uncomfortable half an hour for all of us, but especially for the anesthesiologist. His mission was over. He would return with us to Malta the following day. After the meeting, we all went up to our bedroom, feeling very sorry for the poor guy. He was absolutely mortified. I think he had been so excited to come to a war zone that he had lost any sense that this was really serious stuff—it wasn't a vacation or a gap year trip to be blogged about or put up on Instagram.

The following morning the original team set off to the port with our shamed anesthesiologist. As usual, the roads were crisscrossed with armed rebel checkpoints. The port was still under heavy artillery attack and as we arrived there, we were all too aware of our vulnerability. Only the day before we had had to amputate the leg of a woman who had been injured waiting for a boat to take her and her family to Benghazi. We assembled on the quayside, where a tiny fishing boat was waiting to take us back to Malta. I sat at the stern with my new anesthesiologist friend and, in very calm water, we began moving out of the harbor.

I was both sad and elated. Sad because I had become good friends with some of the surgeons and doctors in Misrata's hospitals, and elated because I felt that for the first time I had used my experience in war and war surgery to train doctors on the ground and to make a difference in their ongoing work. I felt proud that I seemed to have found the leadership qualities to stand on my own two feet and teach. It had also become clear to me that, although my fellow surgeons didn't always speak the same tongue, there was a shared language of surgery through which we could communicate.

As the boat continued to sail out of the harbor the sea grew rougher and rougher, and soon we were again lurching from side to side at almost forty-five degrees. What's more, we were going ever more slowly and were being tossed around while water poured over the sides of the boat. Then, the captain announced that the sea was so rough it had taken off the rudder—he was going to have to steer the boat using the engines on the propellers. Two hours into the journey, we wanted nothing more than to get off the damned boat—even getting caught by Gaddafi's forces would have represented a significant improvement. And after twelve hours, we were all so seasick that death had begun to seem by far the better option.

This went on for another day and night. For a period of at least twenty-four hours, four of us sat in a cabin passing a bucket around, each of us retching so much that I thought we would turn our stomachs inside out. All in all it took us thirty-seven hours to get back to Valletta. When the boat finally docked, we were all unable to walk, and all nine of us came off the boat on our hands and knees clutching anything that could support us. We crawled into the car and crawled out when we got to our hotel. I remember lying in bed holding on to the sides while the room went round and round, occasionally dozing off and hoping that I would never wake up.

My teaching experience in Libya was a catalyst for me to try to put together a training program based on the Definitive Surgical Trauma Skills course that taught all the specialties involved in being a humanitarian surgeon involved in conflict and catastrophes. I had become increasingly aware that surgical training in the developed world was becoming more and more specialized—so specialized, in fact, that I feared surgeons would no longer be able to do humanitarian work. They simply wouldn't have the array of skills necessary to treat the full gamut of injuries a single war surgeon would see in the field.

Specialization in the West seems to become more refined by the year. There are now upper and lower gastrointestinal surgeons, and there are surgeons who specialize only in the mid-gut organs, such as the liver and pancreas. Even in vascular surgery, my own specialty, there are surgeons in the UK who only deal with aortic surgery; those who do lower limb arterial surgery and those who just deal with the veins. Reconstructive surgery, one of the non-acute specialties, is vital in trauma work. Plastic surgeons can transform the futures of patients suffering from congenital deformities such as cleft palate or lip, and fairly simple plastic surgery on war injuries, such as repairing large injuries or covering exposed bone, can help heal wounds that would otherwise get infected. The first time I ever saw the exposed tibia of a patient being covered with a muscle moved from another part of the body was a revelation.

Surgeons dealing with these traumatic injuries also need the confidence to know how to bypass all the clever technical investigations they are used to at home, make the correct clinical decisions, and, if necessary, take the patient straight to the operating room. There is too much reliance on investigations and too little on clinical acumen, due chiefly to the all-consuming fear of litigation. Instilling confidence in the participants was one of the key goals of the DSTS course. We wanted people to be able to make correct decisions based on their own observations, and then to carry out the kind of large and bold incision that was often necessary when dealing with life-threatening injuries.

On my return to London from Libya I had a series of meetings at the Royal College of Surgeons about how best to extend the ideas behind DSTS. The result was Surgical Training for Austere Environments (STAE). The course teaches surgeons how to deal with trauma due to conflicts and catastrophes—without the soothing backup of CT scanners, X-rays, and other state-of-the-art equipment. Sometimes the key lesson is knowing when *not* to do an operation with the limited resources that might be available.

For five highly intensive days, surgeons are drilled in how to treat every region and system in the human body. We cover hemorrhage on the brain, foreign bodies in the skull, fractures of the face, neck injuries including airway problems, chest injuries including how to perform a thoracotomy, and injuries to the heart and lung. Then we look at all the operations required in the abdomen and pelvis, including fractures, and those that fix fractures of the upper and lower limbs. We teach them how to rotate skin and muscle to repair holes in the arms and legs, a vital skill when dealing with severe war wounds. The course ends with obstetrics and gynecology, so that the surgeons are equipped to manage difficult Cesarean sections on their own in the middle of nowhere.

Word soon got out, and the big NGOs began to send us their surgeons—not only first-time volunteers, but many experienced medics who wanted to update and refresh their skills. But even though we—initially, at least—had funding from the Department of International Development and the UK Trauma Registry, the cost of the course—and of getting to and staying in London for it—was pretty prohibitive, which ruled it out for the vast majority of surgeons from poorer or developing countries. I was determined to find a way to change that, too.

- 8 -
RETURN TO SYRIA

In January 2013, a few months after the mission in northern Syria I described in the first chapter, I gave a lecture at the Royal Society of Medicine about the work of Médecins Sans Frontières. It was attended by many Syrian expatriates, some of whom had been busy setting up charities to help their fellow countrymen who hadn't been able to get out. The situation for Syria's civilian population was critical—they were caught up in the fighting and demonized by their own government.

There was a dinner after my talk, and I found myself sitting on the top table next to a man who looked vaguely familiar. Suddenly it came back to me—the last time I'd seen him, we'd been eyeball to eyeball in Hospital Alpha in Atmeh, shouting at each other. It was Mounir Hakimi, the orthopedic registrar from Manchester who was also vice-chairman of Syria Relief. We talked for a long time, and not surprisingly discovered that we had much more in common than that silly argument. I came to understand why he had acted as he had in Atmeh, and he conceded I had had a point too. We parted as friends.

That trip to Syria had made a big impression on me, and as the situation there deteriorated, I knew I had to go back. I contacted MSF in Paris and said I was ready to return—what did they have, where could I go, and when?

To my amazement, however, word came back that there would be no more missions to Syria. In fact there would be no more missions full stop—MSF no longer wanted my services. They operated a strict "two strikes and you're out" policy. The security scare at Alpha, when the jihadis had threatened to overrun the hospital because they'd seen me take photos of the sunset, had been strike two. I had known about the rule not to take any pictures, but, as I have described, everyone routinely ignored it, and MSF seemed quite happy to turn a blind eye to all my priceless training videos, which were technically also in breach of the rule.

And strike one? Well, for that we need to rewind a couple of years, to another mission. But this time, for once, the disaster was natural rather than man-made.

At 4:53 p.m. local time on Tuesday, January 12, 2010, an earthquake measuring 7 on the Richter scale struck the western end of Haiti. The earthquake's epicenter was about fifteen miles west of Haiti's capital, Port-au-Prince, and there were dozens of severe aftershocks. Nearly three-quarters of a million people were directly affected, and estimates of the eventual death toll ranged from 100,000 to over 300,000.

In the chaotic first few days after the disaster the international community began to respond to the calls for humanitarian aid. It had been a bit of a free-for-all, with stories of untrained surgeons performing guillotine amputations on survivors in makeshift clinics. Within a week, MSF had called me to ask if I'd go out there as a general/reconstructive surgeon.

By the time I arrived in Haiti, the majority of life-threatening injuries had been dealt with, but there was a great deal of reconstructive work to be done. I was taken straight to the MSF field hospital in Port-au-Prince and was thrilled to be greeted by Rachel Craven, who had already been there for at least a week and had done a great job in setting up the hospital on the main football pitch. It was a fantastic thing to behold. MSF does the most amazing job in catastrophes like these. Their logistical operation is second to none and their emergency hospital facilities are the best I have ever seen.

The hospital was made up of inflatable tent modules. Each module weighs around 1,200kg and arrives deflated. They are carried from the plane to a truck and then from the truck to the hospital site, ideally somewhere flat. Working nonstop in shifts, it takes around forty-eight hours to construct a whole hospital. Within each tent are long sheets of rubber sewn between huge tubes, with grommets from which to hang room partitions. Once the structure is complete, the rooms inside are converted into operating rooms and recovery rooms, while patients are housed in traditional canvas-and-pole tents nearby.

This tenting concept was developed in 2005 and has been used in the wake of natural disasters all over the world including Pakistan, Indonesia,

Sri Lanka, the Philippines, and Nepal. Working as a surgeon in one of these field hospitals is very similar to operating in any of the best hospitals in the West. And MSF always provides brand-new equipment.

When I got to Port-au-Prince, the hospital had been up and running for a few days and had around 250 patients, many of whom needed further surgery as a result of the rudimentary amputations they'd endured. That first night we were driven back to an expat house opposite Hôtel Le Chandelier, which had been completely destroyed. Standing downwind from it, there was the sickly-sweet scent of death—the bodies of the dead were still trapped beneath the rubble.

For the next three weeks, together with François, the French anesthesiologist I'd been paired with, I performed reconstructive operations, rotating muscles and skin to cover parts of the body that had been badly damaged, often using the latissimus dorsi flap. This is a big muscle on the back, with a single blood supply—if it is isolated and the muscle taken from its bed, it can be rotated to cover most defects in the chest, upper limbs, and shoulder. It is one of plastic surgery's "workhorse" procedures.

But we also took the skin and the radial artery from patients' forearms—swinging it around to cover damage. Most of their injuries were caused by falling masonry. There were plenty of fractures, of course, but many survivors were also suffering from pressure necrosis.

When you press your skin and it blanches, it is because the blood circulating below the skin is driven out. If you're stuck underneath a collapsed building, and can't move, then your skin won't receive any blood and the muscle below will die. This dead muscle then breaks down and minuscule particles enter the bloodstream, eventually blocking the tiny capillaries in the kidney. If this isn't addressed, renal failure and death follow. Maintaining kidney function is therefore one of the first lifesaving maneuvers after rescuing any survivor pulled from a fallen building. It is also why bed-bound patients need to be turned from side to side every few hours, to stop pressure being applied to one particular area of the skin for too long.

We took turns going around all the patients, which sometimes took a whole day. As I was going around the pediatric ward, I noticed a baby who was about six weeks old. She had terrible injuries to her head and right leg, and her right arm had already been amputated. She looked absolutely pitiful. She had been a patient in the city's Trinité Hospital when the hospital collapsed around her—she had been trapped in the debris. It took two days for her cries to be heard.

Apparently, she had had the amputation following her rescue, and it was the rubble in which she had been found that had crushed the top of her head. Miraculously her brain was intact and she appeared cognitively normal—she was responding, drinking milk, and had good bowel and urinary function.

In the residence that night I had a long chat with François. I asked him to come and look at her in the morning and see what he thought, as he was also a pediatric anesthesiologist. So the next day we both trotted off to the pediatric ward and examined the baby properly. I took the dressings off the top of her head and was horrified to see that most of the cranium was exposed—there was no skin over the bone. The cranium itself looked dead, and I feared it wouldn't be too long before she got a life-threatening infection as there was already pus oozing from the wound. I also looked at what was left of her right arm, and found that the humerus was exposed, too. She also had scar tissue all over her thigh, the cause of which was not clear.

François shook his head sadly. He thought she would almost certainly die—the infection would take hold, and meningitis would spread throughout her tiny body. I asked whether there was a neurosurgeon available in Haiti. I was told there was, but he wasn't a pediatric neurosurgeon, and nobody was sure where he was.

It was a desperate situation. And although there were so many children who had serious injuries and who had been made homeless, I couldn't get this little girl out of my head. Knowing that she was likely to die, and that there seemed to be nothing we could do about it, left me feeling impotent and angry.

My concerns about her were compounded by the fact that tensions and rivalries were beginning to surface between the surgeons. With so many of us milling around, all with different degrees of expertise and experience, there was bound to be the odd clinical misdiagnosis. One evening, as I was about to go back to the residence after a shift, I was asked to look at a seven-year-old boy. He had been unwell for several days and had a temperature. He was complaining of significant pain in the right side of his abdomen. When I questioned his father, he told me that the boy's bed was soaked with sweat. There was no doubt it was hot, but the child's sweating was intense. When I examined him his belly was tender, but he also looked slightly jaundiced to me, and I thought the most likely diagnosis was malaria.

Malaria is transmitted by the female *Anopheles* mosquito. Their bites introduce parasites into the patient's blood. They grow within the red blood cells, until they burst out of them to infect yet more red cells. Each time this happens, the patient's temperature rises. They become anemic, and the dead cells begin to block the capillaries in the kidney, liver, and brain. Not only that, there is a significant quantity of other cellular debris which induces a chain reaction of inflammatory cells, which then increases the effect of multi-organ failure. Symptoms may occur at any time, but they usually appear around a week or so after being bitten. It starts with fever and sweating and generally having a flu-like illness, with headache, vomiting, and diarrhea. Symptoms can progress very rapidly in some patients, who can die within a week of diagnosis. Abdominal pain is one symptom of malaria, but it's a fair way down the list. However, there were plenty of other signs that did suggest he had malaria.

There was discussion about my diagnosis among some of the other surgeons, and doubts expressed about whether there was any malaria in Haiti at all. I thought this was a bit much and suggested whoever was on call should do a paracheck. This is a simple blood test that MSF uses all the time. The surgeon on call said he would sort the problem out, although he was pretty certain that the little boy in fact had acute appendicitis.

The next day, François and I were taken to the hospital as usual and began to change into our scrubs. As I put my clothes on the table, I noticed a black bag underneath it. It was a body bag. It was very unusual for there to be a body bag in the changing room, but there it was. I knelt down and unzipped it, and my heart sank. It was the seven-year-old boy, not feverish and sweaty but cold and lifeless. I unzipped the bag further and noticed a surgical dressing in the position where an incision would be made for an appendectomy. François and I marched over to the anesthesiologist and surgeon to ask them exactly what they had found and why they had done the operation. The surgeon said that although the paracheck had been positive for malaria, he had been in no doubt that the boy had a burst appendix.

"And did you find a burst appendix?" I asked.

"It didn't look normal," he said, somewhat unconvincingly. And with that he turned around and walked away.

François let out a volley of French expletives, but what could we do? We would never find out whether the patient did have appendicitis, as there was no pathology laboratory—even state-of-the-art field hospitals hardly ever had postmortem facilities. I am, however, absolutely certain that the mortality risk of operating on a patient with worsening malaria must be extremely high.

I decided to say nothing; it would only have inflamed the situation. The little boy was dead and there was nothing we could do to bring him back. But I vowed that I would not let it happen to anyone else while I was in Haiti. I also decided that, when I got home, I would mention this incident to the MSF hierarchy in Paris. But I never got the chance to do so, as events took a dramatic turn.

I was still preoccupied by the baby girl François and I had examined. In fact, I think everyone on the mission was thinking about her. She had experienced dreadful trauma, was likely an orphan, and had nobody else to look after her. What hope was there for a happy future? Her case seemed to epitomize the tragedy that had beset Haiti. Now, after the boy's pointless death, I became even more fixated on trying to help her.

Urgent plastic surgery to her arm would be a start, so I contacted Waseem Seed, a British plastic surgeon who was working in a hospital near the tennis court a few miles away. I took the baby to see him and he operated on the baby's arm to cover the protruding bone. The operation was a success, but it was only a small part of her rehabilitation.

After Waseem left Haiti, he was replaced by Shehan Hettiaratchy, another plastic surgeon whom I knew from Chelsea and Westminster. I asked Shehan what he thought we should do about the baby's head. His diagnosis was clear: the baby needed to have her cranium removed, then undergo life-preserving surgery to the tissue surrounding the brain. Otherwise, she would die, probably within a week.

A day or so later, I was sitting in the tent wrestling with the problem when I was told there was a British journalist outside who wanted to interview me. His name was Inigo Gilmore. The surname was familiar, and it turned out that his father, Gerry Gilmore, was also a surgeon in London whom I knew very well. Inigo and I struck up an immediate rapport, and he asked me how things were going in the hospital. He had covered the Haiti earthquake almost from the start, and things were now beginning to calm down, so much so that he was only going to be there for a few more days. I told him about the baby girl, and how she had become the focus of everybody's thoughts in the hospital, but that it looked as if she would die soon. He asked if he could see her and so I took him to the pediatric tent, where the little girl had the same effect on him as she had had on me. She stared at him directly with her beautiful, big eyes and I could see his heart melt.

"Is there nothing we can do?"

"I'm afraid not," I replied, "there is nothing in this country that can save her."

That night I went back to the expat house and sat pondering the fate not only of the little girl but of all the other patients I'd dealt with. My time in Haiti was coming to an end; I was due to leave in three days' time. The conversation among the clinicians around the table roamed far and wide about the issues we'd faced, and inevitably the baby's predicament came up. One of the surgeons had the bright idea of drilling holes in her cranium to stimulate granulation tissue, the protective tissue that grows out of wounds to enable healing—one of the body's most miraculous feats of rejuvenation. He was quite right—it is indeed possible that if you drill small holes in bones, granulation tissue may grow. However, it has to be done in live bone, not dead bone, which is what she had. Thinking that she might be needlessly subjected to such a procedure after I had gone horrified me. A cold shiver ran down my spine.

I went to bed determined to save her. I phoned Inigo and Shehan to float the radical idea of taking the baby out of Haiti for the lifesaving treatment she so desperately needed. Shehan suggested I contact Simon Eccles, a plastic surgeon at Chelsea and Westminster, who is a trustee of a charity called Facing the World. This wonderful organization was set up in 2003 by two craniofacial plastic surgeons at Chelsea and Westminster, Norman Waterhouse and Martin Kelly, to treat cranial and facial deformities in patients in the developing world by bringing them to the UK for surgery. In the morning, I contacted Simon and explained the situation. Would he take this poor little girl? Within a few hours he came back to me after speaking to the charity's trustees; he would take her. First, though, Inigo and I had to secure her safe passage out of the country.

There were many hurdles in our way, and we only had around thirty-six hours to make it happen. I discussed the plan with the hospital's project manager. The news that an emergency evacuation was in the cards went around the mission like wildfire. Many thought it was a crazy idea—and it was against all MSF policy to take a patient out of the country. It was OK to move someone internally, but never to take a child out.

There was much discussion that evening among the MSF staff, and emails flew between Port-au-Prince and Paris. Not only that, we learned that there was a new police and customs crackdown on child trafficking to prevent people smuggling children out of the country. We had no backing from the Haitian authorities, the girl had no passport, and we knew nothing about her parents or even for certain whether they were still alive. It felt like an impossible task.

But by now I was filled with unshakeable resolve that this child was going to get out and receive the best surgical treatment available. That meant taking her to the United Kingdom under the auspices of Facing the World. There was a meeting of all the heads of department at the hospital, which I attended. I was told that, while they respected my humanitarianism, if I were to pursue this course I would have to cease being an MSF volunteer in Haiti. I would have to do it as a sole trader. I called Simon Eccles to tell him that I would do all I could to get the baby to London as quickly as possible. Inigo asked if he could cover the story for Channel 4 News. The clock was ticking.

Inigo spent the whole afternoon talking to Haiti's Minister for Foreign Affairs, who finally gave the go-ahead. We still had to find a way of getting the baby out of Port-au-Prince to the airport at Santo Domingo, in the neighboring Dominican Republic. Facing the World agreed to pay all our transport costs and an Aviation Sans Frontières helicopter was organized for the following morning, as were all the plane tickets. But we still had to get her a passport.

After queueing up with hundreds of people in a pen with metal bars at the passport office, I finally got to the front. I sat facing a customs officer and took a deep breath. I wanted a passport to take a six-week-old child with me to the UK. He regarded me impassively. I plowed on, but after about half an hour he said it was impossible and asked me to leave.

"I'm not going anywhere until I have that passport."

"Where are her papers?" he replied. "Where is the photo of the baby?"

He did have a point; I did not have a photo. I rushed out of the office downstairs to find what might well have been the only functioning photocopier in the whole of Haiti. Luckily, I had my camera with me: I called up a digital photograph of her and took a photocopy of it. But it was far too dark; it just wasn't going to work. Screaming that I needed a photocopier, I rushed out of the passport office and made it to a nearby government building. After some pleading and cajoling I photocopied the picture of her on my camera and got the black-and-white picture that I needed.

I ran back to the passport office only to find it was about to close. There was no way they would see me again that day. Yelling like a maniac, I pushed myself right to the front of the line, until I was sitting in front of the customs officer again.

"Here is the photo!" I gasped triumphantly.

He looked at it and said, "OK. Where are the papers?"

I told him I didn't have any papers and with that I was again dismissed. I told him I was not going to leave until I had a passport. Laughing, he beckoned the security guards to take me out. I hung on to my chair, refusing to be moved. Two security guards began wrestling with me, while I clung on to the chair with all the force I could muster and wrapped my leg around the base of his table.

"It is your duty to help this child!" I shouted. "If you don't do this, she will die. How will you face that for the rest of your life knowing that you could have saved her?"

Finally, I had struck a nerve. He waved the security guards away and started lecturing me on how many children he had, what a good father he was, and how he did everything he could for them. He angrily got the necessary forms, filled them in, stapled the picture to a passport, and stamped it.

His last words to me were: "Make sure she lives."

François and I took the little girl by helicopter to the airport, and from there on to Heathrow. We then drove to meet Simon Eccles at Great Ormond Street. Her life was saved, and although there were further twists and turns in her remarkable tale, it's a story for another book. Suffice to say she has turned into a most delightful and beautiful little girl. Her name is Landina.

That, then, was strike one: someone had clearly been genuinely outraged by my flouting of MSF protocols and a black mark had been made in my file. And now they had strike two, the security lapse at Alpha.

I went to the MSF headquarters in Paris to speak to the director of operations in person about their decision not to let me work for them again. I tried to offer a defense on both incidents but was unable to penetrate the wrath directed at me, which felt completely disproportionate.

It reminded me of the time when I was a registrar in Liverpool and had been summoned to see the professor of surgery in his office to be chastised for a fairly minor clinical incident. Professor Sir Robert Shields was a real gentleman, but he ran the department of surgery with an iron fist. I saw senior lecturers go pale and shake with anxiety after being called to his office. I remember standing in front of him, staring into his steely blue eyes, and being quite unable to speak, as all the saliva dried in my mouth. After my admonishment, I walked backward away from his desk, almost bowing as I did so, and fell over the coffee table in the middle of the room, ending up spread-eagled on my back. Whatever soil from his plant pot that had not ended up on my white coat was now all over his floor. The next few minutes seemed like hours as I scooped up the soil in my hands and poured it back into the pot, then positioned it back on the table under the watchful gaze of the nonplussed professor.

My advocacy in Paris got me nowhere. Rules are rules. I would not be allowed to do another mission with MSF. I couldn't believe it and felt very hurt and disappointed. I had given a lot of time and energy to the organization and had promoted their work as much as I could, raising thousands of dollars for them, not least by running the 2007 London Marathon on their behalf. But there it was.

So, if I was to go back to Syria, it wouldn't be with them. What to do?

A few days later, I saw an ad on television for Syria Relief and had an idea. I dug out Mounir Hakimi's card and contacted him to see if I could work with his organization. Our relationship hadn't had the best of starts, but I was delighted that he agreed to take me on. I offered him and several of his Syrian colleagues a place on our inaugural Surgical Training for Austere Environments course. Mounir was very excited that I was going to work with Syria Relief; he felt that many of the surgeons working in Syria at the time needed intensive training.

The five-day STAE course in July 2013 included many of the surgeons with whom I had worked over the years and whom I invited as faculty members to train the delegates. I felt it was important to show as many of the operations I had struggled with over the years as possible, including neurosurgery, faciomaxillary surgery, complex Cesarean sections, and more. Many of the faculty were skeptical because they felt I was teaching things that were well out of the comfort zone of the surgeons participating in the course. However, I am sure that now, as the course reaches its sixth year, they will agree that it is vital to stretch the participants so that they get as much out of it as possible.

That first course successfully completed, I sat down with Mounir and his colleague Ammar Darwish, a surgical registrar from Manchester who had also been on the course. I was to spend a few days at a hospital in a place called Bab al-Hawa, in the north of Syria. They would meet me there, and then we would all travel down to Aleppo together.

Usually, there is no time during a humanitarian mission to feel what it must be like to live somewhere, to understand the surroundings and to begin to love the people you are with. That was all about to change.

They were very kind to me, the people at that hospital. I crossed the Turkey-Syria border on foot, just a month after our meeting in London, and was given an operating room to myself along with a whole surgical team and an anesthesiologist. Most of the work there was to do with nerve reconstruction. I would start operating at around 10:30 in the morning and finish around eight o'clock at night. As usual, people came in to watch me operate. That always makes me nervous, especially if I'm working on something that isn't my chosen field.

Sometimes a patient who has a nerve injury will almost certainly experience loss of movement and sensation in the limb as a result. To treat this, it is sometimes possible to take a superficial nerve from somewhere less important, like the lower leg, and reconstruct the damaged nerve. The sural nerve in the calf is not essential for walking, and the minor loss of sensation in the leg is more than made up for by the restoration of movement. You take the sural nerve and splice it into three or four lengths, putting them together to make what's called a cable graft. But the damaged sections of nerve have to be quite short for the graft to be really successful, and it is almost impossible to know the extent of the damage until you begin the procedure. And when the brachial plexus is damaged, it is even riskier. The brachial plexus is a conglomeration of various nerve roots from the neck, which come together to form nerves such as the median, ulnar, and radial, which supply the arm, forearm, and hand. It looks like a telephone exchange and is very difficult and complicated to repair, requiring specialist help that is really beyond my capabilities. We therefore had to turn away those patients who presented with brachial plexus injuries, although I was happy to take on people with less severe problems, such as median and radial nerve palsies.

In one particular case, though, I found I was struggling to find the median nerve that runs down the arm, as the patient had so much damage in that area. The hospital's orthopedic surgeon was watching, and clearly decided he didn't like what he saw. He scrubbed up rapidly, took the scissors from my hand and started dissecting to find the nerve himself.

I had not asked him for help, and in fact had no clue who he was, except to note that his hair was grayer than mine, as if that were any indicator of seniority. I decided to step back and see if he could do a better job. In the end, he did find the nerve, but it was very close to where I had been working and I'm sure I would have found it there too, if I had been given more time. However, sometimes it's easier to revert to being a significant subordinate, because you really don't know how experienced your more dominant colleague might be. Although I was there in part to teach, there is no point trying to lead all the time—sometimes it's better to try to learn something from the other person. On occasion, though, I have asked for the scissors myself, and more often than not the more dominant surgeon realizes I am not actually a rookie.

As we were finishing the operation, there was an enormous explosion outside, less than a hundred meters from the hospital. Even from well inside the building we could hear windows shattering. There was then an eerie silence, followed immediately by shouting and screaming and the wail of ambulance sirens. I stopped what I was doing and asked the nurse what she thought was happening. She looked extremely nervous, while the orthopedic surgeon pulled off his gown and gloves and disappeared. The nurse and the anesthesiologist then also left—I assumed to see what was going on outside. Soon, the patient and I were alone in the operating room.

After a couple of minutes, I heard another explosion, and more shouting and screaming. It was obvious something serious had happened, and although I began to get that sinking feeling in my chest, as I have many times before, I tried to concentrate on my work. I picked up a suture and quickly started to complete the procedure. As I was doing this, the anesthesiologist came back in and said there had been two suicide bomb attacks and that we had to make space for mass casualties in the operating room.

Around two hundred people had been gathered at a checkpoint next to the hospital. A suicide bomber on a motorcycle had veered into the crowd, stopped, and pulled his detonator. That was the first blast. Of course, people then ran to help the injured, and as more people arrived, a second suicide bomber exploded his vest in the middle of the crowd. This is called a double tap. At the time I had never heard of such a thing, but it is now an increasingly common tactic.

I left the operating room after we transferred the patient onto a gurney and went out to the emergency room. It was a scene of utter carnage. The smell of burning and cordite and gunpowder was overwhelming. The wounded were lying all over the floor and a few were on gurneys. The main injuries were fragmentation wounds to arms, legs, and heads; others were badly burned. Some were propped up against the wall, some were lying down; some were moaning, some were screaming. The majority, though, were silent, shocked. It was difficult to work out who was who, as the whole place was full of people. Most of the helpers were not wearing any kind of medical uniform and I did not know who was trained and who wasn't.

In major incidents with mass casualties we are taught to carry out triage of patients, to determine priority of treatment based on the severity of injury. The word comes from the French verb *trier*, meaning to sift or separate. Patients are normally divided into four categories. P1 (Priority 1) injuries are those that require immediate treatment without which the patient will die because of breathing obstruction or massive hemorrhage. P2 injuries can be delayed for an hour or two before they go to the operating room. P3 are the walking wounded. P4 are the dead or those beyond saving. Clearly, a P1 injury can rapidly become a P4 unless correctly managed.

Having worked with the Red Cross, I was lucky to have trained for this kind of event. It is supposed to work like clockwork—ideally everybody going to a mass-casualty scenario knows exactly what they have to do and what their role is. The triage officer is key; this can be a nurse, a doctor, or anybody who knows how to carry out the primary survey of CABCDE (catastrophic bleeding, airway, and so on).

The role of the triage officer is crucial to the running of a mass casualty. Also, the way that the hospital is organized can have a significant impact on patients' outcomes. The best scenario is where you have one door that admits patients—as they enter, the triage officer gets as much information as possible from each patient's handler or very quickly makes a visual assessment and, quietly and quickly, goes through the steps of the primary survey.

With a bit of experience it takes around thirty seconds to decide whether somebody is in immediate danger of dying from their injuries or whether they will survive for a bit longer. Then, ideally, you will have two separate rooms to send people to: one for P1 and P2 and another for P3 and P4.

In the first room there should be teams of surgeons and doctors and nurses who will provide immediate management of life-threatening injuries. For example, catastrophic hemorrhages will first be treated with tourniquets and pressure to the bleeding area. Airways are then assessed for obstruction and a quick look at the chest to see whether the breathing is equal on both sides. As this is happening, the pulse will be taken.

It's often said that there are different pulse pressures in the radial (arm), femoral (thigh), and carotid (neck) arteries. It is very difficult to know exactly where to feel for these pulses if one is not properly trained. Of them all, the most important is the radial pulse in either arm. If you can feel a radial pulse, then the pressure is around 90 mmHg systolic. This is sufficient to ensure that all the major organs such as the brain, heart, liver, and kidneys will be well supplied with blood. Even if the patient is significantly injured, if he is in this category then he is P2. The P1 injured are those with obvious difficulty in breathing and who do not have a radial pulse pressure. These are the patients who need urgent care and attention, although everyone requires constant review as those who are P2 may suddenly become P1.

Operating rooms are cleared and personnel are allocated so that as many ORs as possible are manned by a surgeon, anesthesiologist, and surgical staff. It takes a lot of extremely careful planning to be able to get the right sort of patient in the right area, so that the appropriate staff can deal with their injury. It may be that operations have to be done on gurneys outside the operating room, but again it is important to provide resuscitation and pain relief to that patient and also have the right surgeon with the right experience.

That's how it *should* work. Of course, nothing like this was happening at Bab al-Hawa that day. Nobody was in charge. Patients were pouring into the emergency room, either dragged in by their feet or carried in by one or two people. Hardly anyone was being brought in on a stretcher. It was pandemonium; the whole place was filled with a cacophony of noise. On top of that, of course, my knowledge of Arabic was very poor and, although I had the training to see what was going wrong, I felt utterly powerless.

It is easy sometimes to become so overloaded by stress that you enter a state of complete paralysis. This has happened to me several times, mostly in my flying career. Once when I was learning to fly the Learjet 45 so many things started to go wrong in the airplane my brain became totally scrambled—there was so much information coming in I found it impossible to assimilate it all and became unable to make even the simplest decision. Luckily, on that day I was in the simulator.

Such inertia usually results from lack of experience and lack of knowledge of the systems involved. It is like everything in life—the more experience and the more practice you have at doing something, the better you will be able to do it.

As I walked around trying to take in the enormity of what had just happened, there were probably sixty people lying on the floor with another twenty or so sitting propped up against the walls of the emergency room. I looked around and tried to think as calmly and clearly as I could about what to do next. I kept repeating the primary survey mantra in my head. "CABC": checking for catastrophic hemorrhage and making sure that there was a tourniquet on an arm or a leg, so we could get control of compressible bleeding; checking the airway, making sure the patient was breathing using both lungs; checking that they had a pulse.

I walked from patient to patient trying to assess the degree of injury. I worked out that the best way for me to communicate with my colleagues was to use my thumb to indicate whether the patient needed urgent treatment or could wait. Many of the patients were beyond help—they had terrible burns that were unsurvivable. The stench of burning flesh was overwhelming. But, despite the horrendous nature of the casualties, the hospital staff were rigorous about the need to be clinically sound and to make decisions based on clinical grounds alone and not emotions. I was hugely impressed by them.

A couple of days later Mounir and Ammar arrived. After an early morning ward round seeing the patients I had operated on, we all met in the hospital canteen. It was seven o'clock in the morning and it was time to set off for Aleppo.

There were quite a few of us in the van, and we were to be accompanied by an escort car that would travel ahead, carrying two men with guns hanging out of the windows to show we weren't to be messed with. Both vehicles had "Aleppo City Medical Council" written on the sides. Inside our car both the driver and his assistant had assault rifles as well. I can't pretend I wasn't anxious—Aleppo was going to be challenging enough in itself, but even getting there felt like running the gauntlet.

The journey took around four hours. It was only about twenty miles and would usually take half an hour. But the regime had blocked the main road and we were obliged to take many detours and side roads along the way. The driver also had to be careful not to make a wrong turn as one mistake would end in certain death—there were roadblocks everywhere, some manned by the regime, others by Islamists whose response to our presence could not be predicted.

Outside the city of Azaz we duly came upon our first barricade. It was a simple affair, just a chain strung across the road like those I'd seen in the Congo and elsewhere. But rather than just the one man policing it, here there were several, and if anything they were even more menacing than those manning checkpoints in Africa had been. They were all dressed in black, with black hoods or scarves with Arabic script across their foreheads, and they were carrying Kalashnikovs with bandoliers of bullets across both shoulders. A cold chill went down my spine as the driver very slightly turned his head toward us, not taking his eyes off the approaching checkpoint, and whispered, "Daesh."

I'd known there were various Islamist groups now operating in the area, but this was the first time I'd heard this name. It was obviously Mounir and Ammar's first encounter with ISIS, too. I was sitting in the back of the car next to Ammar with another Syrian colleague on my left. Mounir and two other Syrians were in front, with the driver and another passenger in front of them. I watched as the windows went down and the barrels of their guns were carefully positioned to show that we were fully armed. Our escort car also wound down its windows to reveal rifle barrels sticking out of the car.

One of the men in black looked through our window and surveyed the passengers in the back. He stared menacingly through the slit in his hood, filling me with quiet horror. I was pinned like a butterfly by his gaze, and acutely conscious of looking different from the others, of not having a beard, and I instinctively leaned forward and put my face against the headrest of the seat in front in an effort to obscure my features. After what felt like an eternity the man made a brief sign for us to move forward and we edged past him.

This was only the first of many such checkpoints, though, and each one we came to seemed to have more men around it, with bigger weapons, and each seemed even more intimidating than the last. I can't remember if it was the fourth or fifth such roadblock we came to when Mounir turned to me and said, "I hope you've got your Pampers on."

Who were these men? In 2012 in Atmeh it had been obvious who was fighting whom: the Free Syrian Army was fighting the regime. But what was going on now? In the coming days I got a better sense of the situation on the ground, and how things had changed since my visit the year before. What I had seen in Atmeh was basically the militarization of the revolution. The armed rebel movements that had emerged later in 2011, as it became clear that peaceful protest against the Assad regime was going to be met with a disproportionate and brutal response, had morphed into the Free Syrian Army. The FSA was initially comprised of soldiers and other security personnel who had defected, but its numbers were soon swelled by civilians who took up arms to defend their towns and villages against the regime.

However, as 2012 progressed, the first cracks began to show. The FSA was in part funded by Qatar and Saudi Arabia, but that money was going to the leader of one particular faction within the FSA, causing friction with other factions who were less well funded. Also, the West was very cautious in its approach to the situation. The Americans promised to supply arms to the FSA but insisted on vetting the groups who'd be receiving the weapons—nervous that high-tech hardware such as anti-aircraft missiles might end up in the hands of extremists. As a result, very few weapons got through, and Assad's warplanes and helicopter gunships could continue to rain down missiles onto civilian areas and rebel bases. The international community also refused to enforce a no-fly zone over the areas of northern Syria held by the rebels.

Assad had pulled a clever trick. In denouncing the protests against him in spring 2011, he claimed they were the work of radical Islamic extremists rather than ordinary Syrians who felt they should have the right to choose their own government. There was a narrative here that he could tap into, as the Muslim Brotherhood had been behind an insurgency against Bashar al-Assad's father, Hafez, in the 1970s. That was effectively extinguished, not least after the massacre of as many as 20,000 people in the city of Hama by the Syrian government. Some of the survivors were thrown into the notorious Sednaya prison, which already housed a number of battle-hardened Syrian jihadis, and left to rot. But in June 2011, on the basis that your enemy's enemy is your friend, many of these people and their sympathizers were released, allowing the regime to claim that the "bad guys" in the civil war were simply the same terrorists that were being fought by security services in the West.

Some of these ex-prisoners and their fellow travelers who had been part of al-Qaeda in Iraq came together in early 2012 to form a new organization called Jabhat al-Nusra. Their goal was not just the overthrow of the Assad regime but the establishment of an Islamic state in Syria. To begin with there was some cooperation between the FSA and al-Nusra, with one observer praising the experienced al-Nusra fighters as being the "elite commando troops" of the FSA. But it was never likely to work in the long term, as the goals of al-Nusra and of more moderate forces in the FSA were fundamentally different.

Meanwhile the Islamic State group over the border in Iraq, now led by Abu Bakr al-Baghdadi, claimed a merger with al-Nusra. The merger was rejected by the other two interested parties, al-Nusra and al-Qaeda, and friction between the Islamist groups intensified. Al-Nusra had strong popular support—they were much less prone to launching indiscriminate terror attacks than the group that soon became ISIS, and more moderate Syrians preferred to focus on the immediate goal of overthrowing Assad rather than the strict Sharia caliphate that would succeed it. This infighting played straight into Assad's hands: rather than facing a democratic, unified opposition pursuing self-determination, he could portray all his enemies as hard-line Islamists.

In May 2013 ISIS took Raqqa, a city about a hundred miles from Aleppo, imposed Sharia law, and began executing Alawites and Christians. Around a quarter of a million people fled, many ending up in camps on the Turkish border. ISIS began to move across northern Syria, pushing out the FSA and al-Nusra, and showing their strength by claiming control of the roads wherever they could. This was what we were seeing on our drive to Aleppo. And the situation was intensifying rapidly—only weeks after we'd been through these checkpoints, Alan Henning was stopped at one of them and kidnapped by ISIS.

As we drove through small villages occupied by Islamic State I thought how strange it must be for the people who'd lived there all their lives—they get up as normal one day, and find that suddenly a bunch of foreigners have taken over, dressed in menacing outfits, carrying heavy machine guns, and driving around in black vehicles with black flags trailing behind them. It was no wonder people were confused about who was fighting whom.

Finally, we were clear of the roadblocks, and there was a collective sigh of relief as we got to a wider, more open road. But we now faced a different danger: the risk of attacks from the air by Syrian jets. This stretch of highway is known as the "death road," and the roadside was littered with the relics of vehicles previously targeted. There was one particularly perilous part of the route where the road was flanked by open fields, providing scant cover, should it have been required, from regime mortar shells or rockets from the Syrian jets circling overhead.

Eventually we approached the suburbs of east Aleppo, the area still in rebel hands, and turned onto Castello Road. This was the only road in and out, along which almost all deliveries were made. The surrounding roads were empty, but as we neared the city it was surprising how relatively normal it still appeared to be, despite being torn in half by the front line of a major war. There was more traffic and many ordinary people trying to go about their business.

But the destruction of this once vibrant, multicultural place, home to some 2.5 million people before the war, soon became painfully obvious. Those buildings not already leveled displayed huge scars, the results of shell and missile strikes. It seemed incredible to me then, and still does today, that Assad's hunger to regain control of his country was such that he seemed quite prepared to ruin it in the process.

We drove on, deep into the ravaged city, at that time probably the most dangerous place in the world. It would be my home for the next six weeks.

-9-

SNIPER CITY

By the time I arrived, in August 2013, the healthcare system of east Aleppo had been forced into the shadows. As I had seen in other countries in crisis, many of the more senior doctors and surgeons had already left—as many as 95 percent of Aleppo's physicians had seen which way the wind was blowing and found a route out. Those who remained were brave and committed, but there were very few of them. In the face of the regime's targeting of healthcare workers and those seeking medical help, one of these courageous doctors had set up a network of secret hospitals to treat people injured in the war.

To escape detection by the regime, he adopted the codename "Dr. White," while his like-minded colleague, Noor, gave the group its name—Light of Life; *noor* in Arabic means light. They recruited several medical students who shared their sympathies with the uprising against Assad, and began carrying out covert medical procedures as well as giving lectures in the basic principles of emergency trauma work. Volunteers would bring wounded protesters to the safe houses, and then leave before Dr. White took over, to preserve his anonymity.

But the care provided was limited, and the risks considerable. Noor himself was kidnapped and later killed, and three of Dr. White's students were abducted by the security forces and murdered. The Light of Life was extinguished, and Dr. White was obliged to change his name again, and become Dr. Abdulaziz.

By this point, some of the now-expatriate Syrian surgeons and doctors had begun to mobilize, setting up charities to try to improve the situation on the ground. My friend and colleague Mounir Hakimi's Syria Relief was one of them. Aid and ambulances were making their way into Syria from Turkey, but the approach was scattershot. Supplies would arrive at a clinic that had just received a truckload of medicine, while other facilities were completely overlooked.

A more coordinated response was urgently needed and so Dr. Abdulaziz set up the Aleppo City Medical Council (ACMC). The plan was to establish a formal network of clinics across the rebel-held eastern half of the city. These clinics were also assigned code names, which initially ran sequentially from M1 to M8, but later hospitals were given random numbers to disguise how many there really were. The subterfuge did not stop there—ambulances and other medical vehicles carried no sirens, insignia, or logos, and at night drove with their headlights off. Anything that looked like help for the injured was, according to the regime, aiding the rebels and so in their eyes a legitimate target.

Our first stop on arriving in Aleppo was one of these hospitals, M10, where we were greeted by the surgeon in charge, who would become a great friend. Dr. Abu Mohammadain was in his late thirties, a urologist by training—and a very good one. The other doctors there were more junior, and needed a lot of help to deal with the number of casualties with gunshot wounds. We were taken to a small room that served as the canteen and were given a wonderful welcome meal of hummus, olives, fresh cucumber, and tomatoes, followed by some delicious tea. Dr. Mohammadain showed me the pockmarks on the walls from a recent rocket attack, and advised me to sit near the door and not the window.

We left M10 to continue our journey to M1, the hospital where I would be based. It was a little bit farther south, and closer to the front line. As we drove through east Aleppo, I asked our driver about the mounds of rocks I could see everywhere along the route. It turned out that they had been put there deliberately to shield civilians from sniper fire from the western half of the city, which was still mostly controlled by the regime. There were also two badly damaged buses, one on top of the other, to provide further protection in an area that had been turned into a market. The market itself was full of people, with lots of fresh fruit and vegetables on display in many of the stalls. There were shops open, too, and I was amazed to see hundreds of people on the streets simply going about their everyday lives while the conflict raged around them.

But it was plain that life for civilians in Aleppo was already appallingly difficult, whether in the rebel-controlled east of the city or in the government-controlled west. I later learned that the rebels were trying to encircle the western side of the city and close the main road up from the south. This was the primary inbound route for food and other supplies, so the regime was—equally desperately—trying to keep it open, though without much success. There was very little fresh food reaching the people of western Aleppo, and the only way to get any was to cross to the east, where supplies were more plentiful. At first, the front line was dotted with passageways allowing access to and fro, but gradually these were closed off until only one major entry-point remained, the Karaj al-Hajez crossing. At one point, around 10,000 people per day were heading from the west to the east in search of food.

To make things even more difficult, all the people going back and forth every day to shop, work, attend school, or simply visit relatives risked the wrath of both sides. Residents from the west might face harassment or even kidnapping for ransom when entering the rebel side, or be arrested when they tried to return home. It was worth the risk, though. In western Aleppo a loaf of bread cost 300 Syrian pounds, but only 65 in the east. These poor civilians caught between the rebels and government soldiers also faced snipers positioned in the city hall, or other nearby buildings. Dozens of people at the Karaj al-Hajez crossing were shot at by snipers every day. But people had to eat.

As we pulled up outside M1, about a hundred meters from the crossing, we piled out of the van with our bags and cases. I had my big gray suitcase with me, which always looked incongruous in a war zone. The first thing I noticed was the armed guards at the door, but they wore smiles as well as guns and greeted us warmly. I had expected to be shown inside and then be given a welcome tour, but the moment I arrived I was asked to help with an operation. I changed quickly and was shown into the OR, where I was greeted by a man with a beautiful command of English who looked completely at home in his environment.

"We've been waiting for you!" he said jovially. This, it turned out, was the famous Dr. Abdulaziz.

On the table was a man who had obviously been shot. It looked like the bullet had traversed his bowel, and he needed a small bowel resection to join it back together. It was a bit of a baptism of fire—I hardly had time to take in my surroundings before Dr. Abdulaziz told me to scrub up at the small sink nearby. I was handed a surgical gown made of green cloth rather than the usual disposable paper version that I was used to in the UK. The gloves were also different, and quite difficult to put on as they were thin and easily torn. Once I was ready, Dr. Abdulaziz handed me a pair of scissors and forceps. "The case is yours," he said. "This is the eighth procedure I've done today and I need a break. But I'll assist you."

And then came a sudden flashback to that disastrous test flight for Astreus a decade earlier—I was wearing the wrong glasses again. My operating glasses were in the big gray case, along with my gas mask, loupes, and other equipment. I couldn't now take off my gown and gloves and make my excuses—a man needing an operation was on the table in front of me and there were four other surgeons in the room, including Ammar and Mounir, all waiting to watch the English doctor join up two ends of a small bowel.

I squinted as hard as I could to try to focus on the bowel and explained that I was going to make a connection called a single-layer anastomosis. I took the 2-0 Vicryl suture and prayed to God that I would be able to see what I was stitching it to. It wasn't the best anastomosis ever, but it was successful, although I think Dr. Abdulaziz noted my shaking hands. The anxiety about operating this quite simple procedure in front of my new colleagues was overwhelming.

Afterward Abdulaziz introduced me to everyone, and we had a chance to talk about the plight of Aleppo and its people and what the ACMC was doing to help. He told me his parents and the rest of his family lived in west Aleppo—he had to be very careful to hide his real name, as if it became known that he was working on the east side his family would have been killed immediately.

The doctors at M1 were all very young, mostly in their mid-twenties. There was Abu Abdullah, the general surgeon; Abu Hozaifa, the vascular surgeon; Abu Waseem, the plastic surgeon; and Abu Khalid, the orthopedic surgeon. Each of the other trauma hospitals I worked in while I was in Aleppo—M2, near the old city, and M10—had only general surgeons. The specialists would go from hospital to hospital when and if required.

As a result, I shuttled between the hospitals constantly, driven around by a wonderful man called Abo Abdo, who carried a Kalashnikov on his dashboard to show he wasn't to be messed with. However, even though many of the doctors had a title to indicate their specialty, they were still basically trainees with very little experience, and there was much work to be done to fill the gaps in their knowledge and train them up to be as effective as possible, as quickly as possible.

In M1 the majority of injuries we saw were gunshot wounds sustained while traversing from one side of the city to the other. There were as many as seventy individual snipers dotted around east Aleppo at that time. They simply picked people off as they were crossing the street, going to work or going to the shops. Abdulaziz told me that I should expect that anyone and everyone who came in would have been shot by a sniper—from babies to the elderly, no one was immune.

As Abdulaziz filled me in I marveled at how buoyant and enthusiastic he seemed, after all that he had been through. I warmed to him immediately, and I was, in fact, already feeling very comfortable with all my new colleagues. It was still light, and after chatting for a while we decided to go for a walk outside the hospital. We went around the back of the building so I could see the effects of the airstrikes.

I found myself looking at an apartment block that had been cut in half. One side had been demolished and lay in a pile of rubble, but the other half was still standing, exposed to the world like a giant doll's house. You could see right into the apartments, full of beautiful wooden furniture, and in some cases ornaments and figurines were still standing on the tables and dressers. One apartment had a kitchen with wooden spoons, pots and pans, and bottles of oil and other condiments ready for use. It was the most bizarre snapshot of obviously well-to-do lives that had been torn asunder.

Abdulaziz posed for a photograph with me and Ammar. In it, I can see that I look sad, but Abdulaziz is smiling, apparently full of hope for a better future.

Ammar was my roommate, along with one of the junior surgeons. It turned out that Ammar had contacted Syria Relief to see if he could stay with me

24/7, acting as my interpreter, minder, surgical student, and confidant. I soon realized how lucky I was to have a man of such integrity by my side, willing to defend and support me unconditionally throughout my time in Syria. He had a terrific sense of humor, too, which also proved invaluable. Over the weeks that we spent together I came to depend upon and trust him completely. We became so close that I regarded him not just as a friend but as the brother I never had.

Wherever I went, Ammar went, too. On the rare occasions when I was out of his sight, he still knew exactly where I was. Missions can be rather isolating and solitary experiences, so this was a novelty, but I soon came to appreciate deeply his reassuring presence.

I was excited that first night, spent trying to sleep on a plastic mattress without sheets in my surgical scrubs, which I barely took off for the next six weeks. I already felt a strong affinity for the people I'd met, reinforced by my instinctive sympathy for the ordinary people of Aleppo and what they were going through. I had my USB drive, too, with the STAE course on it, and felt confident I'd be able to do more here than save only the lives of those casualties put in front of me.

We didn't have long to wait. Around five o'clock the next morning, we heard the first of many *tap-tap-taps* on our door—could we come down to one of the operating rooms straightaway? Ammar and I found Abu Abdullah in the middle of a procedure. He apologized for getting us up so early—"Usually," he said jokingly, "it doesn't start until around eleven o'clock, when the snipers get out of bed."

We went to scrub up in the small square room along the hallway that served all three operating rooms. The patient was a man with, as ever, a gunshot wound—a tricky one in that the bullet had traversed and almost split the right lobe of the liver in two. The patient had lost quite a lot of blood before coming in, and Abu Abdullah was trying to do the operation on his own. I told him I'd be happy to assist but he said he wanted to learn, and handed me his scissors and forceps.

As often happens, I shuffled through my memory banks, reliving the many times I had previously operated on injured livers. The first thing to do, I told him, was to compress the liver back to its normal anatomy. Do this for as long as it takes the bleeding to stop, and for the anesthesiologist to catch up with fluids. Very often surgeons forget that there are people at the top of the table struggling to maintain the patient's blood pressure and pulse, and continue to operate without letting the anesthesiologist know what's happening.

We squeezed on the liver for about half an hour, taking it in turns—me, then Ammar, then Abu Abdullah. After an hour or so, though, it was obvious that it wasn't working. I suggested we use the omentum to try to stop the bleeding. This is a big, fatty, apron-like membrane in the gut, which can be wrapped around inflamed organs to seal them off—hence its nickname "the policeman of the abdomen." Abdullah had never seen this done and it gave me great pleasure to show him how to move the membrane and roll it around the liver. Once attached to the liver, we closed up. Two hours later the bleeding had stopped, the patient was in recovery, and we could go back to bed.

A few hours later we resurfaced to join other members of the hospital—doctors, nurses, and ancillary staff—for breakfast. Looking around the room, I saw about forty people eating and chatting together, like a huge family—a family in which I felt entirely at home. The women ate separately, in a room downstairs, except for one of the paramedics, Um Ibrahim. She also acted as a kind of liaison officer between the hospital and the various FSA groups in the area. A formidable woman, loud and funny, she didn't take any nonsense from anyone and she effectively ran the hospital. She was ably assisted by her delightful fourteen-year-old son, Ibrahim, who helped keep everything running smoothly. She was wonderful, a mother figure to everybody in the hospital. She would come into our bedrooms to make sure we were all OK, she would be in the emergency room helping with casualties, and she would even pop up in the operating room to see how things were going.

She came up to me during that first breakfast.

"How many children do you have?" she asked. I said I was sorry, but unfortunately I didn't have any.

"Oh. How many wives do you have?" she said. I smiled and said, "None, Um Ibrahim."

"*Whaaat!*" she said, laughing and shouting at the same time. From then on, at every meal we shared, she would engineer an opportunity to say, "I am going to find you a wife before you leave Aleppo."

Just as Abu Abdullah had predicted, things began to get going at around midday, when the first gunshot wound arrived at the hospital. The emergency room was at ground level, as were the somewhat battered X-ray machine and the three ORs, which were run by Mahmoud, the operating room manager. He was very experienced and was completely at ease with all the equipment that we needed. Surgeons would simply shout out his name and he would run to get the equipment they wanted. He was no pushover, though—he would stand his ground and shout back if he thought the request was ridiculous.

The emergency room was run by a tall, good-looking young man who had been in his third year at Aleppo medical school when the revolution started. After six months in charge, he had become extremely adept at identifying which patients needed immediate treatment by examination alone. I was amazed that he managed the emergency room with just four trained nurses and ancillary staff. The ancillaries were men and women who had given up their jobs—as shopkeepers, tailors, factory workers—and were being trained to become emergency nurses.

It was difficult for me to show my face in the emergency room, though, since it was rather more public than the operating rooms. Security was paramount, as Ammar kept reminding me. There were armed extremist groups roaming around, including members of ISIS, whose base in the Qadi Askar district was just a short distance from where we were working. It was vital that I kept a low profile—I was almost certainly the only Westerner in Aleppo at the time, and it would have been a major coup if I had been kidnapped. I was confined to the hospital grounds, leaving only to go to one of the other hospitals; I therefore spent most of my time in the operating room.

Only once did we make a mistake, driving from M10 back to M1 with a new driver. He took a shortcut down a road we usually avoided, and we found ourselves approaching the ISIS headquarters with its black flags flying from the rooftop and black-clad armed guards at the door. Ammar was first to realize the driver's error. It was too late to stop and reverse, as that would have attracted too much attention. Thinking quickly, he yelled at me to get down as we approached the building and as I slipped out of sight he told the driver to step on it. It was a close shave—the headquarters had become a prison and place of torture for many of Aleppo's civilians. There were also rumors that one of the MSF surgeons working in Aleppo province had been taken there for questioning and subsequently murdered.

There was an ever-present threat, and I had to remind myself continually not to become complacent. Abdulaziz told me that in November 2012 he had welcomed the British orthopedic surgeon Abbas Khan, who wanted to help at M1. The day after he arrived he was seen leaving the hospital with his camera. He told the security guards out front that he was going for a walk. Apparently, he wandered down a road and directly into the hands of the government forces.

After he was reported missing his mother moved heaven and earth to try to locate him, and he was eventually found in a prison in Damascus, thanks to unofficial assistance from the Indian and Russian embassies. All attempts to get him released failed and then, thirteen months later, the UK coroner's court deemed that he had been murdered by the Syrian regime in December 2013. The authorities denied this, claiming that he had hanged himself, but nobody believed them.

Abbas Khan was married and had two children. I have since met his entire family, including his mother, who is still in a state of shock and disbelief that this could have happened. More recently, I gave the inaugural Abbas Khan Memorial Lecture at King's College London, where he had been a medical student. His name, at least, lives on.

On that first day alone in M1 eleven civilians shot by snipers were brought in. One of the commonest causes of death from gunshot wounds is exsanguination—massive bleeding. Survival often depends on how quickly the patient can be transferred after the sound of the gunshot has faded. Working at M1, which was so close to the Karaj al-Hajez crossing, we could hear the shots, and the wounded usually took only five or ten minutes to reach us.

Some were not so lucky, though. Once a sniper had opened fire, the crowds would understandably scatter for cover, often leaving the injured party lying in the middle of the road. It was very dangerous to then go to that person's aid, as whoever did so would also become a target. It seemed to me utterly bizarre that government snipers could sit in a hotel room on their own side and shoot civilians in cold blood simply to stop them from getting food. But the regime's justification still applied: any civilian crossing to rebel-held eastern Aleppo was considered a terrorist.

The doctors at M1 told me they had been losing a lot of patients to gunshot wounds to the major arteries; they needed significant training. I immediately agreed to give evening lectures, plus hands-on instruction for any surgeons who wanted it, where I could show my "best moves"—introducing them to new techniques, or little tricks such as how to hold their hands or instruments to save time on the table.

On that first day, all eleven patients who had been shot survived—but only after a solid eighteen-hour shift at the end of which I fell onto my bed absolutely exhausted.

We were woken early the next morning by the sound of Syrian jets flying over the hospital. I was too tired to move, but it wasn't long before the *tap-tap* on the door. When we got to the operating room a boy of about fifteen was being given external cardiac massage while being prepped for surgery. The anesthesiologist at the top of the table only looked a year or two older than the patient—but he had intubated him and was now putting lines for fluid access into the subclavian vein. Looking at the heart monitor I saw what looked like an agonal rhythm, an abnormal electrical pulse in the heart indicating imminent death.

There was a large, deep wound on the front of the boy's chest, and several more on his abdomen and legs. He had obviously suffered the impact of a missile or shell, being injured by fragments either from the bomb itself or from flying masonry or other debris.

I watched for a second or two while one of the young surgeons poured iodine over the boy's abdomen and prepared him for surgery. He made a long incision from the chest right down to the pubis, but his colleague was still performing external cardiac massage and this movement forced his guts out of his abdomen, rather like squeezing toothpaste from a tube. There was no abdominal bleeding. It was almost as if the incision was a default, rather than a course of action based on the evidence. I quickly checked the boy's head, neck, and legs, all of which seemed normal. He was still being given cardiac massage, so it was difficult to determine what was wrong. I suspected that, with the chest wound overlying his heart, the injury was to the heart itself and was probably a condition called cardiac tamponade.

The heart lies in a tight fibrous bag—the pericardial sac—that surrounds and protects it. Any direct injury fills the sac with blood, and the resulting pressure impairs the organ's ability to pump—this is cardiac tamponade. What follows is potentially catastrophic: the venous pressure goes up and the arterial pressure drops. If you were to listen with a stethoscope you would hear muffled heart sounds rather than a strong beat.

If I was right and the boy did have a cardiac tamponade then he was in the final stages—his heart was so compressed that it had stopped beating. I was certain he needed a thoracotomy—opening up the chest to cut into the pericardial sac, first to relieve the pressure and then to allow access to the heart itself. But I needed to tread carefully. I had only just arrived, they didn't know me from Adam. If I was to intervene, I had to be right, and it had to be at the right moment. The other surgeons needed to see that if something wasn't done, the boy would die.

Through Ammar, I asked respectfully if I could show them something. They agreed and Ammar went to the opposite side of the operating table as I took up the scalpel. I made an incision just below the nipple, following the course of the ribs as I cut through all the intercostal muscles as quickly as I could. I then got the two other surgeons to pull the chest open. I scooped the boy's lung up with my left hand and then Ammar took over, which freed me up to make a longitudinal cut into the pericardial sac. With that, the blood that had been packed in under huge pressure poured out and the heart that had stopped beating came back to life.

I asked Ammar for a large chest retractor and everyone in OR shouted "Mahmoud!" Within seconds he was back with a Finochietto retractor. This is a rack-and-pinion-type device which spreads the ribs and keeps them locked open, giving the surgeon clear access.

Looking around, there were now about ten surgeons in the operating room. No one had ever seen this type of procedure before. Very quickly, I isolated a large bleeding point on the front of the right ventricle due to the fragment from the bomb, which had been pouring blood into the pericardial sac. I guided Ammar's finger over the hole in tune with the heart's beating, and then cut a small piece of the pericardial sac and used it as a protector for the stitch. Within about ten minutes the bleeding had stopped, the heart was beating properly and the ECG trace was normal. It was a small miracle. We had caught this boy just in time: another few minutes and it would have been too late; his brain would have been starved of oxygen.

It also came at the right time for me, in terms of my mission in Aleppo. A fairly routine diagnostic process for me was revelatory for the Syrian surgeons. They had never seen anything like it. For this to have happened on only my second day cemented my authority and convinced them from the beginning that there was a lot they could still learn. You could see it was a revelation for them, and there would be others like it. Arriving as a volunteer in a new hospital, in a highly charged situation, is very delicate. You have to acknowledge that you are a stranger, an interloper, and of course sometimes people don't take kindly to having their authority challenged, or there might be cultural differences to overcome. You need to establish trust, but also to radiate authority. I always tried to show humility, saying "Please can I just show you something?" or "Would you mind if we tried this a different way?" Sometimes I had to be more assertive, especially if I encountered resistance and the patient was in real danger, but very often the local doctors realized that they had reached the limits of their knowledge or experience and were grateful for the intervention.

Word of the heart operation quickly spread, and that evening I discussed the case with what seemed like every surgeon left in Aleppo, who had all congregated for a debriefing session. I began to hold these sessions every day to discuss the patients we'd operated on, the reasons why we had chosen the procedures we'd carried out, and the results that we expected. I used the STAE information from my USB drive and Ammar and Mounir would take turns translating my lectures. We felt that an hour a day was enough—everyone was tired and needed rest as well as education.

Later, Ammar and I went to see the boy in the intensive care unit. The door was locked, so we knocked and a nurse let us in. I was expecting to find more colleagues inside, but was amazed to see four beds all occupied by ventilated patients and no other staff. The small room had syringe drivers containing drugs on a stand, and high-tech monitoring equipment measuring arterial blood pressure. There were charts at the bottom of each bed which the single nurse was very carefully completing with all the relevant observations including pulse, blood pressure, temperature, urine output, all the outputs from all the drains, the quantities of drugs that were being infused, as well as the oxygenation of the ventilators. There was also a small arterial blood-gas machine to measure the oxygenation of the blood.

How was it possible that such a high-tech environment could be run by a solitary nurse? The nurse smiled and gestured to two cameras pointing at each patient—one to monitor the patient himself, the other to observe the charts. The nurse told us that these were fed by Skype directly into the intensive care unit in one of the hospitals in Washington, DC, where there was a Syrian-American ICU specialist looking at the monitors twenty-four hours a day, and adjusting the patient's medication and ventilation based on the clinical parameters. Not just at our hospital, either. All the intensive care units in Aleppo were linked into the same American hospital. It was an amazing system, beautifully managed by an ICU specialist called Ammar Zacharia, who had trained all the ICU nurses so they knew exactly how to respond to the comments of the online specialists.

We continued to monitor the boy for the next twenty-four hours, until he was well enough to breathe on his own. His parents were ecstatic, and it was a wonderful way to kick-start my mission.

Some days were busier than others, and some were so busy that the days merged into the nights and vice-versa. We didn't see many fragmentation wounds that autumn, but the gunshot casualties kept coming; Aleppo was sniper city. I remarked to Abdulaziz that on some days there was a weird consistency to the injuries we saw coming in—the patients all seemed to have been shot in the same part of the body. One day we would receive patients who had all been shot in the left groin area; on other days six or seven would arrive who had been shot in the right groin. The same thing was happening with patients shot in the upper limbs and chest—the injuries all seemed to be on the same side, in clusters. Also, despite the snipers having telescopic sights, we rarely saw the head shots that would have resulted in an instant kill—the goal seemed to be to wound, to disfigure or disable. Abdulaziz told me that he'd heard that the snipers were playing a game: they were being given rewards, such as packs of cigarettes, for scoring hits on specific parts of the anatomy. He was certain this was true, and certainly the evidence seemed undeniable.

This sick competition reached its lowest point toward the end of my time there when it appeared that one particularly vicious and inhumane sniper had a new target of choice: pregnant women. One such casualty arrived in M2, shot in the abdomen. The bullet had missed the baby but gone through the placenta. The woman was on the operating table only a few minutes after being shot and we delivered her baby boy via a lower segment incision, but the placenta had been completely shattered and had stopped supplying oxygen to the fetus. I quickly clamped the cord and gave the infant to one of the nurses to resuscitate, but sadly she was unable to do so. We carefully sewed up the mother's uterus in the hope that she would be able to have another baby; we weren't going to let the sniper take that away from her.

The same day another sniper's victim came into the hospital. She was a first-time mother, almost at full term, and had been due to be admitted for a breech delivery or an elective C-section, depending on how the labor progressed. She was very beautiful, wearing an immaculate white headscarf and a long, elegant coat that now had a large red stain on the front. There was a bit of confusion among the emergency staff as, although obviously distraught, she seemed well. For some reason she was sent for an abdominal X-ray. The X-ray showed that the bullet was still inside her abdomen, but appeared also to show, horrifically, that it was lodged in her unborn baby's head. The woman was immediately transferred to the operating room.

The sniper must have taken aim when she was standing sideways on, as the entry wound went through the widest part of her belly. We performed a midline incision as quickly as possible and I saw there was a gaping hole through one side of her uterus. An incision was made in the lower segment and we pulled the baby out. It was handed to a nurse as usual but it was pointless: the poor thing had a massive head wound and was obviously dead. The uterus by this time was in tatters and we ended up having to give the mother a hysterectomy as well. She survived, and there is no doubt we made the right decisions to try to save her and her baby. But at what cost? She had lost her one and only child, and she would have to live with the knowledge that she would never bear another. This was probably the most upsetting and shocking act of violence I had ever witnessed against another human being. And by this time, I had seen a few. I was determined to try to publicize the horror of what was going on in Aleppo when I got back to London.

A few days later, Ammar and I were grabbing an afternoon nap between operations when there was another knock on the door. A patient on the ward was going into shock—a chest drain that had been put in a couple of hours earlier was filling up with blood, and Abu Abdullah wanted to know whether I could help him with a thoracotomy. I said I'd be there in a few minutes.

I dragged myself out of my slippery plastic bed and put on my operating shoes, which by this time were caked in dried blood—the floor was often awash with it. Once I got to the OR Abu Abdullah talked me through a right-sided chest injury—the man had been shot in the back just below his shoulder blade. There was much debate about whether or not we should put him in the crucifix position and perform a clamshell procedure—that is, opening both sides of his chest and lifting it up like the hood of a car—or whether we should put him on his side and just operate on the right chest. Abu Abdullah wanted to put him on his side, as he wanted me to teach him a posterolateral thoracotomy. This is not the standard teaching in trauma, but I figured it would be easy enough to reposition him if we needed to and convert the incision into a clamshell.

The patient was very pale under his thick beard and it was obvious that he was bleeding significantly from the chest wound. The anesthesiologist put him to sleep and even put a double lumen tube down, so that we could deflate one lung while ventilating the other—that was how good these young anesthesiology technicians were. We positioned him on his left side, cleaned him, and draped him. I stood in front of the patient with Ammar by my side. I handed the knife to Abu Abdullah and showed him where to make the incision, from just below the right nipple all the way around underneath the shoulder blade to the back.

By this time, the eastern side of the city was almost entirely surrounded by the regime. However, the Aleppo City Medical Council still managed to smuggle medical supplies in and out, usually strapped to the back of motorcycles that were fast enough. We'd just had delivered a device called a cutting diathermy, brought on the back of one of these bikes like a pizza, and we used it to cut through the fascia and the muscle until we got down to the ribs. I told Abu Abdullah to cut on to the sixth rib and to push the tissues aside so that we could enter the lung.

As we did so, blood began to pour out of the chest cavity. I asked the anesthesiologist to try to reduce the airflow into the lung so we could see what was going on. Dividing the inferior pulmonary ligament allowed us to see that the lower right lobe had been completely destroyed, and there was significant bleeding from the pulmonary vein.

This is a very difficult operation at the best of times, with a very high mortality rate—the same injury had caused the death of Princess Diana. I told Abu Abdullah that, if he wanted, I would stitch the hole in the vein and he could then do the lobectomy. Ammar very stealthily used the aspirator so I could see where the hole was in the vein, while Abu Abdullah moved the lung out of the way and used his fingers to staunch the hemorrhage.

Just as I was about to suture the pulmonary vein, the doors of the operating room burst open. I looked up to my right and could not believe my eyes as I saw six fully armed men wearing black combat fatigues and headscarves storm into the room. They were obviously ISIS fighters, and the patient on the table was one of them.

My heart lurched and I froze stock-still—only my eyes moved as I searched out Ammar's gaze, wide-eyed like me above his surgical mask. *Oh*, I thought, *so this is how it ends*. I felt a rush of adrenaline and I turned away, looking down at the floor. I could hear them doing something to their weapons, either putting in new magazines or playing with the safety catch. I looked around again, and as I did this, I caught Ammar's eye once more—he shook his head almost imperceptibly—*No, don't say a word, leave this to me.* The leader of the group came forward with his gun leveled at us.

"This is my brother!" he said aggressively, in English but with a very strong Russian-sounding accent. Not just ISIS, but Chechen ISIS. "What are you doing to him?"

In English, Abu Abdullah told him that we were trying to save the man's life, but we did not know who he was.

"You should have asked us before taking our brother to surgery!" was the reply. "Who are these people?" he went on, indicating Ammar and me.

Abu Abdullah told him that we were the two surgeons. It was obvious that the man wanted me to speak, but Ammar piped up in his strongest Syrian accent to say that we were all surgeons simply trying to save the man's life.

By this time I had begun to shake. It was all I could do to keep my legs from buckling under me. I felt as helpless as I had been at that Congo checkpoint—I was literally trembling with fear.

"Who's this?" he said, pointing to me, and with this he started to walk around the table.

Abu Abdullah whispered in my ear, "Don't say a word," before turning back to the ISIS leader and saying, "This is the senior surgeon. The senior surgeon is stopping your brother's bleeding and must not be disturbed. If you disturb him, he will not be able to save your brother's life."

The leader came up to the operating table and peered into the man's wound to see what we were doing. The rest of the group milled around the room menacingly—a few sat on the floor while others leaned on equipment and made themselves comfortable. By this point, I was the very opposite of comfortable—it was now very difficult for me to proceed with this complex and delicate operation because I was shaking so much. For the first time in a very long time I decided to pray.

I am not religious, but there have been times when I have felt the need to turn to a higher being. It's like tuning a radio—without warning, I suddenly need to change the frequency from my current waveband to the waveband that allows me to talk to God. It is hard to describe; it's as if moments of acute intensity propel me to a different level of consciousness. This was one of them.

I prayed that God would allow me to complete the operation. I asked him to control my shaking hands, which were still pressing on the wound. I wanted to start stitching but I could not open my mouth to speak. I tried gesturing to Ammar and he guessed, correctly, saying "Suture, suture!" but I was given the wrong one and I had to try again. And then an extraordinary thing happened—as I looked down to what I was doing, very anxious that there had been a hiatus in the operation and that the ISIS leader would start wondering what was going on, I felt Ammar's head gently touch mine, in a simple act of brotherly love. Suddenly, my hands relaxed. My legs were still shaking, and my body still rippled with tension, but my hands were steady.

It took us another hour to finish the operation. I sutured the hole in the pulmonary vein in complete silence. Usually, there is a lot of banter in the operating room when we're doing tricky maneuvers, but today we were silent apart from an occasional quiet comment in Arabic between Ammar and Abu Abdullah.

As we neared the end we heard gunfire outside, and a walkie-talkie that one of the men was carrying crackled into life. He went out of the operating room and was soon followed by the others, apart from the leader, who stayed with us right until the final suture was in place and he had satisfied himself that the bleeding had stopped. Then he too left.

The patient had been exceptionally lucky—he had been shot through the lung, and had been hosing blood, but ironically, because his ISIS comrades had burst into the OR, I had spent more time simply pressing my trembling hands onto his wound and when I was at last able to take my hands away I could see where the hole was.

Afterward, I found myself feeling confused and a bit lost. I had saved the man's life in the most difficult circumstances and I suppose it was lucky for me, too—if he'd died, the inevitable questions would undoubtedly have revealed my identity. I am sure that if the ISIS commander had known that I was a British subject he would have killed me on the spot. My dilemma was that I had, once again, saved the life of someone who might go on to commit terrible crimes. Did that make me complicit somehow? This time, I had known exactly who my patient was and could make an educated guess about the kinds of things he had done or might do. And yet, I still firmly believe that it was my duty to save his life. As on that occasion in Pakistan, in the back of my mind I hoped that one day he might find out that the doctor who had helped him was a Christian with no feelings of prejudice or hate toward him.

Meanwhile, terrible crimes were being committed every single day. A few weeks after this incident, at M1, an ISIS fighter recovering on the ward had a religious disagreement with another patient who had fractured both his legs in a bomb blast. That evening, the same group of Chechen ISIS fighters, who were renowned for being sadistic and vicious, stormed into the hospital, went up to the ward and dragged the man with the fractured legs down the stairs. Once outside the hospital, they stabbed him to death in the middle of the road then cut off his head in front of hospital staff and civilians passing by. They had thought that he was a regime soldier, but in fact they were wrong; he was a member of the Free Syrian Army. But it was too late for apologies. The cracks between the rebel factions were beginning to show, and the mood in Aleppo was turning against ISIS.

Another story Ammar told me struck a particular chord. Apparently, a German doctor had visited the hospital in Azaz, near the Turkish border, which was treating both ISIS and FSA fighters. For some reason the doctor had taken a photograph of one of the ISIS fighters he had operated on. The jihadist took exception to this and demanded the camera. The doctor was ushered out of the ward. More ISIS fighters arrived, saying they wanted to take not just the camera but the doctor, too. But the FSA, who were guarding the hospital, refused to allow him to leave.

Outside the hospital, ISIS opened fire and killed two of the FSA guards. This then sparked intense fighting in the hospital, which subsequently spread throughout the whole town. Eventually, the FSA had to abandon the town altogether, leaving it under strict ISIS rule.

Four things had come out of this, according to Ammar. First, any Westerner in Syria was now viewed as a spy and, if caught, would be subject to severe punishment. The second was that it made no difference if the Westerner was a doctor. Third, it might now be very difficult to get back to Turkey, as the only road between Aleppo and the border passed through ISIS territory; and, finally, it was a disaster for the Free Syrian Army. They were supposed to be fighting Assad's regime but were now also fighting a rival rebel group bent on creating its own caliphate.

I had reached a point at which it became increasingly difficult to carry on as normal. If I had thought too hard about what was going on around me, I would not have been able to function. From then on, every morning, I prayed, asking God to keep me safe so I could do my job. I concentrated on the patients, on training my colleagues, and spending as much time with them as I possibly could. It seemed the only sane response in this insane war.

That said, I didn't feel particularly at risk in Aleppo—I was surrounded by people I now considered friends. None of us knew how things would play out. Many of the moderate Syrians I worked with didn't really know who ISIS were; their mind-set was still that of Syria before the revolution. They were used to dealing with all religions and cultures in their city, and had very little time for extremism. They all still thought that the West would come to their rescue and provide the Free Syrian Army with all the weapons and equipment it needed to topple the regime.

The work went on, and after a month or so I began to feel that I was really making a difference to the doctors, surgeons, and nurses working there. But, as ever, it sometimes felt like one step forward, two steps back. One particular case vividly demonstrates this.

Two young boys who had been shot in the leg were admitted to M1. Both had huge, pulsating swellings in the mid-part of their thigh. Listening through the stethoscope, I could hear the characteristic hum of an arterio-venous fistula—a connection between the artery and the vein caused by the bullet, very similar to the boy who had been injured in the neck and whom I had treated in Bosnia all those years ago. Without treatment they would develop heart failure.

I operated on the first boy with Abdulaziz. After controlling the blood vessels above and below the injury, we opened up the swelling. Blood immediately poured out of it. We disconnected the artery from the vein and repaired all the holes in the blood vessels. The patient recovered well and left the hospital two days later.

The other boy was about fifteen and he, too, had a fistula with a large false aneurysm in the middle of his thigh. Abdulaziz, who had really benefited from my lessons in vascular surgery, thought we should take him to M10, so that the surgeons there could also learn some of these techniques. We set off in the back of Abo Abdo's ambulance, with the patient smiling at me in pleasant anticipation of having his leg fixed and being free of pain.

When we arrived at M10 I gave the team a short briefing on what we would be doing and how I was going to do it. His hemoglobin was fairly low, and as this was to be an arterial operation I suggested that we should have some blood available. One of the nurses took a sample to determine his blood group. By the time the boy was anesthetized, there were five or six surgeons including Ammar scrubbed up at the operating table.

I carefully made the incision on the boy's thigh and isolated both the vein and artery above and below the lump. We had a discussion about anticoagulation, and the need to prevent thrombosis from occurring when clamping blood vessels. I asked for 5,000 units of the blood-thinner heparin to be given, and we waited for a couple of minutes for the drug to circulate around the body. I then applied the clamps and gave the knife to one of the other surgeons, asking him to make the cut into the large blood vessel. This he did with enthusiasm, but unfortunately while he did so he knocked off one of the small clamps on the artery, which fell to the floor, and arterial blood pumped out. We had only two clamps and the other was on the lower end of the artery. Panic took over as we tried to occlude the artery before he bled too much. He had lost about a liter of blood in the space of a few minutes and I asked for a unit to be brought up from the "blood bank," which was an old Coca-Cola machine. There was never enough blood—perhaps only a couple of units of each type.

While I was waiting, I decided to take the long saphenous vein from the boy's other leg to use as a bypass across the aneurysm on the injured leg. That done, we were still waiting for the bag of blood and we continued to wait for what seemed like a very long time. Eventually, it arrived and was put into the intravenous line.

About half an hour later things started to go wrong. The boy began to bleed from every cut surface—not just the leg with the aneurysm, but also from the other leg where I had removed the superficial vein. I couldn't understand it. I asked our anesthesiologist, who was a very obliging senior colleague, about the heparin—perhaps he had given 50,000 units rather than 5,000? He showed me the bottle to confirm that he had given the right dose. On the operating table things started to go from bad to worse; the boy was now pouring blood from every capillary we touched. It was like a horror film; everything was bleeding. He needed additional transfusion and very quickly. The calm, controlled atmosphere of the teaching operation had become one of those surgical nightmares in which everything starts to go wrong and very quickly spirals out of control.

We were now seven hours into an operation that usually takes a maximum of two, and still I could not control the bleeding. Eventually, we finished. Although the operation was technically successful, it had been an unpleasant experience for everyone. Ammar and I went down to speak to the boy's father, who was remarkably calm. He told us that he had lost his other two sons in the same attack, and that he was sure God would protect his only surviving child.

Exhausted, we went to bed but I woke early and waited for Ammar to wake up, too. I was anxious to go and see the boy. At eight o'clock Ammar and I set off from M1 to M10 and went directly through to the intensive care unit. It was a terrible sight. Our patient was blue and cyanosed. He was so ill that he did not have the strength to pull off his oxygen mask. He was in complete renal failure and was producing no urine—what was in the urine bag was dark, concentrated and almost black. I examined him and was horrified to find that even the intravenous line that he was lying on had caused a line of bruising on his skin. What on earth had happened? I sat and racked my brain and it was Ammar who came up with the possibility that he may have had a transfusion reaction—he must have been transfused with blood from the wrong blood group.

I was stunned. I went down to the OR to see if I could find the blood grouping card.

We all fall into one of four blood groups: A, B, AB, or O. If you are blood group A, then you have a protein attached to your red cells called A-antigen (an antigen is a molecule that can induce an immune response, or antibody). Group B has the B-antigen, blood group AB has both the A- and B-antigens, and blood group O has neither antigen attached.

The blood that circulates through the heart, arteries, capillaries, and veins carries nutrients and oxygen to the body's cells, and removes carbon dioxide and intracellular digestive products. Blood consists of plasma, containing the microscopically visible elements of the blood, the erythrocytes or red blood cells, the leucocytes or white blood cells, and the platelets. The platelets aid in the coagulation process and stop bleeding from wounds. The white blood cells combat infectious diseases—the so-called immune response. In addition to carrying around these cells, the plasma contains antibodies, which attack and destroy antigens. There are particular antibodies to particular antigens. In the case of blood transfusion, if the patient is group O, there are no antigens on the surface of the blood cell, so you can transfuse type O blood into any patient because the new blood will not be attacked. It is for this reason that Group O is called the "universal donor" and is stocked in most blood-bank fridges to give patients in emergencies.

However, if a type-O person receives a blood transfusion from any of the A, B, or AB blood groups, then the antibodies in his or her plasma will attack the antigens on the surface of those red cells and cause those red cells to stick together and subsequently burst. The bursting effect of the red cells releases not only hemoglobin but also many other compounds, which tend to consume all the clotting proteins in the body. They produce micro-clotting, which then blocks off the capillaries in various organs such as the liver and kidneys. This is called disseminated intravascular coagulation, and is very bad news.

There is an easy way to determine a patient's blood group using a card which already contains antibodies in three small discs. Disc one contains A-antibody, disc two contains B-antibody, and disc three contains a rhesus positive or negative antibody. By placing a drop of blood onto each of these discs, we can establish the patient's blood group. A patient who is blood group A will see agglutination, or clumping of the red cells, in the first disc (antibody A), but nothing will happen on disc two, and the blood will remain in solution. Checking which disc contains agglutinated blood tells us the blood type.

I took Ammar with me to confirm the boy's name in Arabic. We searched through the bins from the night before, which, thankfully, had not yet been emptied. After an hour or so we found his card. His blood had been dropped onto the disc containing the antibodies and all the discs were in solution, indicating that he was blood group O rhesus negative. We checked to see what blood he had been given. To my horror, he had been given two units of blood group AB. I realized that whoever had checked the blood had been confused into thinking that agglutination meant that the blood was *compatible* rather than being incompatible. This also explained the delay—the technician hadn't been sure exactly what he was looking at.

The poor boy had been subjected to the worst transfusion reaction possible. Not only had he been given two units of AB blood, this was followed by several units of O blood. If he had only been given O blood, then he would have been OK, and not now suffering the effects of the so-called ABO incompatibility, which caused the uncontrollable bleeding.

I was extremely disturbed that such a simple mistake had led to him dying in front of my eyes, and I felt entirely responsible. If I had not been there, he would not have had the operation, and he would not have died, as he did a short time later. The pain that I could see in his father's eyes was awful to behold, and although Ammar spoke to him in Arabic all I could do was hold his hand and watch him break down in tears, but with unbearable dignity. We drove back to M1 in complete silence. I went to our room and, while Ammar tried his best to console me, telling me it wasn't my fault, I cried my eyes out.

I think my reaction was a combination of everything that was wrong in this dreadful war. Young people being shot by ruthless snipers, and inexperienced hospital staff trying to do their best in very difficult circumstances, but sometimes making fundamental mistakes that cost lives. I felt so bad that I thought I should go home—the weight of this disaster was too much for me. If this had happened in the United Kingdom it would have resulted in a prolonged court case, perhaps even a manslaughter charge, and someone would have gone to prison. There are many checks in the National Health Service to stop things like this from happening, but at home and around the world there are many cases of human error leading to fatalities. Being in a war zone does not absolve us of responsibility. I shall carry that guilt with me for as long as I live.

Ammar's response was to say that if I did go home he would return with me, but he emphasized that our job was actually to stay in Aleppo and to treat as many wounded people as we could. It was a learning experience for everybody concerned. It's just a terrible pity that sometimes the learning has to come from such dreadful mistakes, mistakes that are tattooed onto our psyche.

Despite the tragedies there was real progress. I had by now become very close to all the surgeons and was really enjoying their company and the camaraderie. As with Libya, it was an agreeable change to be able to work with and teach local surgeons rather than other expat volunteers. We lived together, ate together, and worked together. There was genuine harmony in all the operating rooms and I found myself turning into something of a mentor, even a father figure, given how much older I was than most of my colleagues. They would call at all hours of the day and night and Abo Abdo, one hand on the steering wheel while holding a cigarette with the other, an AK-47 propped up with his thigh, would drive us at breakneck speed, blasting the horn in his ambulance from hospital to hospital, room to room, where sometimes I would operate and sometimes just give advice on what to do next. We grew more and more ambitious, and patients who in most war zones would be merely patched up were offered major surgery.

The surgeons got better and better at managing the arterial and venous wounds from gunshots, and also vastly improved their understanding of damage control surgery, buying their patients more time by stabilizing them and keeping them warm before plunging into a big procedure. Most of the immediately lifesaving operations took maybe forty-five minutes or an hour, rather than tying up the OR for hours with an operation the patient might not have been robust enough to survive. Then, when there was a lull, we could return the stabilized patient to the OR and do the procedure in a more controlled, less stressful environment. It was a much more efficient way of doing things and the doctors quickly saw the benefits. Soon enough, patients no longer routinely died after a significant trauma, and it became quite rare for anyone to die. Indeed, almost unbelievably, in a three-week period in September 2013 throughout the whole of Aleppo not one patient who made it to hospital died of a gunshot wound.

We became so bold that when a fourteen-year-old boy who had been shot in the abdomen was brought to M1, Abu Abdullah and I decided to risk an extremely tricky procedure—and all the other surgeons were there to watch. A bullet had gone through the boy's duodenum and the head of the pancreas, which it surrounds, and also destroyed the right kidney. This part of the duodenum contains both the common bile duct and the pancreatic duct, which together are called the "ampulla of Vater," after Abraham Vater, the German anatomist who first described it in 1720.

The pancreas produces not only insulin but also the enzymes that go into the duodenum to help digest food. If the ampulla of Vater is destroyed, then pancreatic juices leave the duct and digest all the surrounding tissue. Bile will also seep out and inflame things further. The bottom line is that if the ampulla of Vater is destroyed the patient will die, unless a heroic operation called a Whipple procedure is performed.

Abu Abdullah turned to me and said, "How about it?"

The pancreatic duodenal complex is one of the most difficult areas in the body to deal with, especially if it has been disrupted by trauma. Despite aggressive surgical intervention, even in high-volume trauma centers patients will suffer a high rate of complications, long intensive-care stays, and a mortality of around 50 percent. However, if we left this boy alone it was 100 percent certain that he would die.

Luckily it was fairly quiet that day. I asked Abu Abdullah how much blood we had left. "Probably around ten units," he replied. I had not done a trauma Whipple operation before; the last time I had performed a Whipple procedure was for cancer of the head of the pancreas about twenty years earlier. Before we started, I checked my computer to see if I had the operation saved on my hard drive. Fortunately, I had once taken copies of photographs of the Whipple procedure from Cameron's *Atlas of Surgery*, and there they were. I looked over the steps several times. It involved removing the head of the pancreas, duodenum, stomach, and bile ducts and joining up what was left in an anatomical spaghetti junction with many joins. If any one of the joins leaked, he would die. The operation took eight hours to perform and slowly news got out that we were doing it. The operating room slowly filled up with many surgeons coming to watch and learn.

After all the joins had been performed, we were left with a very swollen bowel, which was impossible to get back into the abdomen. I had modified a procedure used to repair incisional hernias called a component separation, where one of the three muscles in the side of the abdomen is divided to provide more give in the anterior abdominal wall. This allows the wall to be stretched up to 7cm on one side, and if performed on the other side as well, you can buy up to 14cm more space. I have used it many times—it's an excellent technique and we used it now. Amazingly, all went well. We clapped and cheered as the patient was moved from the operating table to the gurney to take him upstairs to the intensive care unit.

The following day Ammar and I went with some trepidation to see whether the patient had survived the night. To our relief and delight the boy was sitting up in bed, asking if he could have a drink. Two days later, he left the intensive care unit and went back to the general surgical ward, and by the next day he was devouring a bowl of hummus and bread. We were able to remove his drains and send him home on day six. Incredibly, a boy with a 100 percent mortality risk a week earlier became the only person in Aleppo to have had a trauma Whipple operation, and we could claim a 100 percent success record for one of the most complex surgical procedures in the book.

By now I was also running my own outpatients' clinic at M1, in a small room isolated from the rest of the emergency room so no one could see me entering and exiting. I would sit there for a few hours in the morning with Ammar, and patients would be brought to us having survived all manner of traumatic wounds.

A lot of them needed reconstructive surgery, so I was pleased that the plastic surgeon, Abu Waseem, seemed keen to learn as much from me as he could. There were patients who had suffered significant injuries to their arms and legs, leaving exposed bone, and others with huge defects in their skin and muscle that needed proper covering.

Abu Waseem had just finished his basic surgical training and was desperate to be known as a plastic surgeon. He had seen a lot of operations but had not done a huge number himself, and with the bulk of our work being plain trauma surgery there wasn't much scope for him to get his teeth into "plastics" apart from helping the odd burn victim. I decided to take him under my wing and suggested that if there was any reconstructive work I'd be happy to take him through it.

Amid all the carnage of the gunshot wounds we were dealing with on a regular basis, usually between twelve and fifteen cases a day, the people of Aleppo were still trying to go about their normal routines. However, equipment broke down, machines stopped working, and improvisation was often necessary. There was an engineer in the neighborhood with his own lathe, and he repaired broken-down cars using bits of metal that he managed to scavenge. He was so good that he was working around the clock to keep the transport system of east Aleppo running. One day his lathe broke down and he put both hands into the machinery to tighten a nut deep inside. He must have nudged a switch because the lathe started and his left hand was ripped off above the wrist and his right hand was mangled.

I was having a cup of coffee on the top floor of M1 looking out on the street below when I saw a car come screeching to a halt. Out came the engineer, running to the hospital with both arms pouring blood. I rushed downstairs and into the operating room. We quickly applied a tourniquet to his upper arms to stop the bleeding but he was in so much pain that the kindest thing to do was to anesthetize him immediately. Once he was safely under, we assessed his wounds. His left arm was so badly damaged he needed to have his forearm amputated. His right hand, his dominant hand, needed saving. He still had his thumb and index finger and half of the middle finger, but the rest was gone, including half the forearm.

Abu Waseem and I amputated his left forearm and then carefully debrided what remained of his right hand. Because of the tissue loss and the exposed bones and tendons, he would definitely require covering, but not right then. We needed to take it slowly: dress the wounds and get rid of any infection that might take hold by bringing him back to the operating room several times, removing more dead tissue each time while also giving him antibiotics. Over the next few days he got stronger, and his right hand had some movement in the thumb and forefinger. It was time to cover the wounds.

I asked Abu Waseem if he had ever done a groin flap. This is where you redeploy a flap of skin from the groin, slightly larger than the palm and fingers of a large hand. The flap is supplied by a small artery coming off the femoral artery. If you raise the flap, still based on its artery, you can cover the damaged hand by securing it into position over the groin. Once the flap is in the right place and is sutured to the remains of the hand, it is then left in that position for around three to four weeks until the blood supply from the hand provides circulation to the flap, at which point the flap can be separated from the groin to allow the whole hand to be covered in skin.

I could see the delight on Abu Waseem's face. He was finally going to do a major plastic surgery procedure. With about fifteen other surgeons from Aleppo watching, I took him through the groin-flap process. It took a while, but it was a great pleasure to watch him dissect and carefully mobilize the flap. Because of the nature of the engineer's wound we had to use external orthopedic fixation devices on his pelvis and remaining forearm to fix the hand and arm in place so they couldn't move.

There is a special sense of achievement when a junior surgeon carries out a difficult operation under the watchful eye of a senior colleague. It is hard to put into words, but I could see that Abu Waseem was euphoric. No matter what had come before, no matter what he had seen, the fact that he had performed this operation well gave him great pride and confidence in the future.

It was now mid-October, and I was coming to the end of my time in Aleppo. Ammar decided to stay on for another three months, but said he would accompany me back to Turkey before returning to the city. On the night before I left the whole hospital threw a leaving party for me. Everyone I had worked with in Aleppo came to M1, and music and fun and laughter and dancing went on through the night.

The next morning all the doctors lined up early to see me off. At the end of my last hug I said a very tearful goodbye but promised them that I would come back. With Dr. Mohammadain driving, Ammar and I then set off in convoy, up Castello Road toward the north, and the border at Atmeh. On the way I couldn't help thinking what an amazing adventure I had just had. The young doctors and surgeons I had worked with were perhaps the most remarkable group of individuals I had ever met. I had trained several of them in their chosen specialties. Abu Hozaifa had become adept at treating most of the arterial injuries and was able to perform all the techniques available to improve the blood supply and avoid amputation. Abdulaziz became a thoracic and cardiac surgeon, able to open people's chests and stitch hearts when necessary. Abu Abdullah became the most proficient and best general surgeon in Aleppo. Abu Waseem went on to expand his reconstructive repertoire. There were many others, of course, too many to mention, but all of them were a joy to teach and I was really impressed with their skills. And these surgeons went on to teach other surgeons, and so the circle of learning continued.

All was going well with our journey until we reached a ten-mile section of road that traversed the area controlled by ISIS. By this time, we were fully aware of what was going on with the extremists. A couple of miles before we reached Azaz, the ISIS stronghold, one of the tires on our van burst. We all piled out of the car and our armed escort positioned themselves nearby, scouting the area. Luckily there was a spare in the trunk, but there was no jack. Without much thought to the precariousness of the situation, six of us grabbed hold of the vehicle and raised it bodily, while Dr. Mohammadain attempted to change the tire.

Suddenly Ammar told me to get back into the car. A pickup truck with a big black flag fluttering from the back was coming toward us. I crept into one side of our car as the vehicle full of armed ISIS fighters drew up on the other. I peered over the bottom of the window to see one of them beginning to question Dr. Mohammadain about what we were doing there. Ammar quickly came to the car and whispered to me to hide. I duly slipped down onto the floor in the back and tried to pull the foot mats and anything else I could find over me, terrified. Then I felt a judder as the car slipped—with fewer hands to hold it up, it had fallen. Fortunately, Dr. Mohammadain was not badly injured and it drew the attention of the ISIS gang from the rest of the car. They did not bother to check it. I continued to hide for about an hour until the wheel was changed and we could move on, making it safely to the Atmeh border crossing just before it was due to close.

The sense of relief at crossing back into Turkey was immense. I was struck again by how on one side of a barbed-wire fence there was tranquility and normality, while on the other there was a full-scale civil war. Just two hours later, Ammar and I were having a Turkish bath in a comfortable hotel as if nothing had ever happened. We hugged goodbye before he left on his return journey to Aleppo, and I said I'd see him again soon. I was sure I would be back.

– 10 –
LIFELINE

I returned home with mixed emotions. On the one hand I felt exhilarated, and strangely optimistic about the future in Syria. I had a feeling that the extreme fundamentalism of ISIS would not take root there and was still expecting that more would be done by the international community. And I was happy to have played a part in training and teaching those brave surgeons who would carry on helping the people of that desperate country.

But there was anger, too, at the manifest injustices of the conflict, and how ordinary civilians with no ax to grind were being targeted by their own government. Yes, it was confusing that those opposing the regime were a hodgepodge of conflicting interests, from moderate pro-democracy campaigners to hard-line Islamists. But the children? How did they fit in to the paradigm that if you aren't with us, you're against us?

I had resolved to share the dreadful story of the pregnant woman whose unborn baby had been shot, and Mounir was also keen for me to go on television and talk about how bad things were in northern Syria. Being inexperienced in the ways of the media, though, I made the mistake of allowing the TV news item to focus on the wrong thing: I mentioned the sick game the snipers were playing, and that they were being rewarded for hitting particular parts of the body on different days. And so, of course, that became the story—not the plight of the victims, or the horrendous number of casualties, but the snipers' game. I felt sorry for Mounir too, as I didn't really have the chance in the interview to discuss the work of Syria Relief, which was doing more for Syrian civilians on the ground than any other organization.

A few days after that, I was interviewed by *The Times* newspaper. I wanted to raise the issue of civilians being targeted, and do it in the right way. I was mindful also of the power of an image over even the most compelling testimony, and thought about the photos and videos that I'd amassed for training purposes. Among them is an X-ray of the pregnant woman's near-full-term fetus, clearly showing the bullet lodged in its head. It remains one of the most shocking images I have seen.

I discussed the story with the *Times* journalist and then with Mounir. Perhaps we should publish the X-ray—it was so profoundly distressing it might startle the world into paying attention to what was happening in Aleppo, and put pressure on the United Nations to try to stop the war. As I was working for Syria Relief, I felt it was up to them to agree, which they did. The picture was published on the front page of *The Times* in October 2013 with the headline "Assad's snipers target unborn babies."

I was glad the story could be told, but again it rather sensationalized the war, and the real message of how bad the situation was for civilians in Aleppo took second place. Not only that, there was then a debate about the picture's authenticity. Even though I also had a photograph of the baby after we had delivered it from its mother's uterus, showing the entry wound in the skull, more was written about whether the picture was real or fake, and whether I was telling the truth, than about the fate of the people of Aleppo.

I didn't give up, though. Some weeks later I was invited on the BBC's *HARDtalk* program, to be interviewed by Stephen Sackur. This time I was given the opportunity to talk in more detail about what was going on. I tried to convey what it was like to be on the front line, dealing with significant casualties every day; the difficulty of trying to keep patients alive without the materials and backup we were used to at home. Our discussion ranged far and wide and I talked about the need to set up humanitarian corridors, policed by the UN, to supply aid and food to the civilians who were being cut off and besieged by the Syrian regime—or, indeed, by the rebels. It was my fear that the country could become one of the worst humanitarian disasters the world had ever seen. Of course there were—and, sadly, are still—no easy answers, but it was good for once to be able to talk about the real problems Syria faced.

A couple of weeks later I was invited by Syria Relief to a big fundraising dinner. To my astonishment I was the main attraction for the evening. Never in a million years did I think that I would end up signing autographs for dozens of people. There was a poignant video produced by my Syrian colleagues of my work there, including many heartfelt words of thanks from patients and doctors. I truly felt that they loved me, and I loved them.

But amid the feelings of pride and satisfaction, I felt adrift. I had returned to my usual NHS work straightaway, as I almost always do—I rarely took any time off after a mission, finding it easier just to get straight back to work.

I carried on, but something was awry. I had had an extraordinary experience in Aleppo; my presence had made a very clear and discernible difference, both while I was there and in the teaching legacy I had left behind. In London, there were any number of people who could carry out the operations I was doing, and do them just as well if not better. In the UK I might save one person's life a month, whereas in Syria it had been ten a day. What the hell was I doing here?

Home for me at that time was fairly spartan—the same small flat overlooking the River Thames opposite the London heliport. I had no family, my parents had both died several years before, and I had no other ties, no girlfriend. I was quite short on cash, having sacrificed a lot of income to do my overseas work. I was disillusioned, bereft even. There was nobody I particularly wanted to be with, and I realized I never felt so alive as I did on a mission, or so fulfilled in my job at home as I was abroad. I began seriously to consider packing in my NHS work in London and going overseas full-time. This was not pure altruism—I knew that part of the appeal was the selfish pursuit of the thing I wanted to do, and the excitement of risk.

It was also harder and harder to adjust to life back in London, and the first-world problems I had to deal with—sometimes I just wanted to shout at people, "Get over yourself! You think you've got problems?"

Christmas 2013 was pretty miserable. I had actually hoped to avoid it altogether, having answered a call from the ICRC to help out urgently in the sectarian violence between Christians and Muslims that had broken out in Bangui, in the Central African Republic. But it was a shambles. I was to fly to the CAR via Paris, but the weather was awful. On Christmas Eve the winds were howling at gale force, and that we made it to Charles de Gaulle Airport at all was testimony to the skill of the pilot.

We landed in France at around two in the morning on Christmas Day, and I prepared to spend the night on a seat in the departure lounge to await my connecting flight at 9:00 a.m. An official laughed at my plan, saying no planes would be taking off the following morning, so I booked myself in to a hotel close to the airport and decided to drown my sorrows with the help of a well-stocked minibar. I fell into unconsciousness at around four in the morning, but was woken a few hours later by the sound of airplanes taking off. The weather front must have blown through, or perhaps the wind was going straight down the runway. I chiseled my tongue from the roof of my mouth and ran down to the Air France check-in desk. I was too late, the woman said, to board the Bangui flight. I told her that I was working for the Red Cross and implored her to let me board the airplane—I could see that the gate was still open. But with magnificent Gallic aloofness, I was dismissed and told I would have to wait for the next flight—in a week's time. No matter how strongly I remonstrated, she would not let me on the plane.

I telephoned Harald Veen, the head surgeon for the Red Cross, and offered my sincere apologies for the mishap. I then booked a flight later that day to Douala, the largest city in Cameroon, where I ended up some sixteen hours later. I knew that there was a service from Douala into Bangui, but stupidly hadn't confirmed that it was still running. When I got to Douala, the fighting in Bangui had escalated, and so many people were taking refuge in and around the airport that all incoming flights had been canceled. The situation was liable to change at any time, though, and I was advised to wait in the transit lounge in case it did.

So there I waited, for four days of the Christmas holidays, staring at a man sitting on a plastic chair staring at me sitting on a plastic chair. There were only the two of us there in the transit lounge while everybody else went off to have fun. He seemed extremely interested in me, fixing me with a gimlet gaze while endlessly chewing betel nut. I tried to strike up a conversation but he couldn't speak English or French (or Welsh), and I couldn't speak Bantu. He just stared.

By December 29 I could take it no more, and boarded a plane to Paris and from there to London. I arrived feeling rather sorry for myself, but I was just in time to listen to the broadcast of another interview I'd done, this time for BBC Radio 4 with Eddie Mair.

I had been a bit uncertain about this request—I respected Eddie Mair as a journalist and radio presenter and worried that I wouldn't meet his expectations. I'd heard him maul a few politicians on air—who probably deserved it—but I worried he might similarly tear me apart. So it was with some trepidation that I had cycled off to meet him in his lion's den at the BBC a fortnight earlier—and could not have been made to feel more at home. It was another way of getting the message out there about what was really happening in Syria.

I was also able to tell listeners the story behind an image that was constantly in my head. One day I'd seen a boy of about fifteen who had been shot in the chest and was lying dead on a gurney in the emergency room. His thick black hair was immaculately groomed, and although he was dead, he seemed to be smiling from ear to ear. During a particularly frenetic time, with many patients being brought in, I kept looking at this boy's face, sometimes unable to concentrate on what I was doing. Why was he smiling? Was it because the pain of what he or his family had been through was now over? Or was he laughing at the pure insanity of the situation we all found ourselves in? I will never know, but that smiling boy's face still peers at me through the darkness of sleepless nights.

Later in the spring I did make it to Bangui. By then the most intense fighting was over, and there were only sporadic outbreaks. There were quite a few cases that required further intervention, and I spent much of my time there re-operating on many unfortunate surgical complications. But there were some fascinating cases on the ward, for example a man with classical tetanus. In Britain it is found only in medical textbooks, but here was a man who had an injury through which the bacteria *Clostridium tetani* had entered his bloodstream and caused his muscles to go into tetanic spasm. Any sudden movement of a muscle group can cause that muscle group and the groups around it to spasm. The medical term for facial tetany is "risus sardonicus," which produces the characteristic sardonic grin. It can be fatal: if the respiratory muscles go into spasm some patients may become hypoxic and die. The treatment was simply to wait and see, while administering antispasmodics and sedation.

Apart from the sporadic clashes outside the hospital, most of the fighting I had to deal with was internecine, among the expats. Sometimes you are with a fantastic group of people and they all work together as a team. Sometimes . . . not so much. When a young man was admitted with a gunshot wound to his thigh—the bullet had gone through the superficial femoral artery and vein—there was no doubt that he needed an operation, otherwise he would lose his leg. It was a fairly straightforward procedure that involves taking control of the artery and vein and then dissecting out the damaged section, and bypassing it using either a vein from the other leg or a vein patch.

However, the anesthesiologist, who was also an expat, refused to put the patient to sleep because she didn't agree with what I was going to do. As I have observed before, we're all allowed to disagree, and I have no problems in discussing difficult cases. But the anesthesiologist was outraged, refused to listen to any reasoned arguments, and just stood in front of me, shouting. I controlled myself with great difficulty and found another anesthesiologist. But even then I could hear the first anesthesiologist bending somebody's ear about it in the next room. It was all very unpleasant, and even in the morning, when the boy was recovering from a successful operation, she was still muttering about it and radiated disdain for me during the ward round. She told me it was a silly operation: the boy should have had a primary amputation and she would be proved right in the long term. The boy left hospital three days later with all his limbs intact.

Oddly, given the severely testing situations I have found myself in, it is such moments of conflict with colleagues that are among the most stressful. Incidents like this eat into me, constantly playing on my mind. It's not that one person is right and one is wrong; in human behavior sometimes there is simply no resolution. The anesthesiologist still felt I had done the wrong operation when we discussed it around the table days later. On short missions like this, team dynamics are crucial, and this kind of friction can destroy the smooth functioning of the unit. Her point was that infections are rife in this part of the world, and if the graft had become infected, the boy might indeed have had to lose his leg. But that is not a reason to perform a primary amputation and ruin a patient's life forever. For the rest of the mission, we neither spoke nor worked together, avoiding one another on the hospital halls like children in the playground.

I came back from the Central African Republic at the beginning of May 2014. It had been rewarding to help people, as ever, but the antagonism had soured the experience and I realized I'd also been frustrated by not being able to do any teaching—I'd been working with other international volunteers, not locals.

I resumed my NHS work once more, but was so busy I had no time to think about myself. I was still running the Definitive Surgical Trauma Skills course at the Royal College of Surgeons and had also run another Surgical Training for Austere Environments course before going to Africa. I had another couple of months to prepare for the next STAE course in August, and there was talk of my returning later in the year to Syria with Syria Relief. Life was full—but also somehow empty.

The wonders of the smartphone allowed me to cycle around London listening to music or the radio. The BBC's *Today* program was a must in the mornings, and I tried not to miss *PM* as well. Listening to the morning and evening news bulletins, there was no doubt that things were beginning to heat up again in the Middle East, with further conflict looming between the Israelis and the Palestinians.

There had been a significant deterioration in living conditions in the Gaza Strip since mid-2013, following the shutdown of illegal tunnels connecting Gaza with Egypt, its neighbor to the south. Hamas, though regarded as a terrorist organization by Israel and the US, had been elected to power in Gaza in 2006 and were using these tunnels to smuggle weapons, building supplies, fuel, and consumer goods past the sea and land blockade of Gaza that the Israeli government had imposed since its assumption of power in the area. After the decline of the Muslim Brotherhood in Egypt, the Egyptian military had also clamped down on the tunnels, concerned that equipment from Gaza was going to Islamic militia operating in the northern Sinai Peninsula, who had killed dozens of Egyptian policemen and soldiers.

This had a huge chain reaction in Gaza: loss of fuel supplies forced its only power station to shut down, causing serious problems.

In late April 2014, nine months of US-mediated peace talks collapsed. In May, two Palestinian teenagers were killed in the West Bank over clashes with Israeli troops. On June 12, three Israeli teenagers were abducted (and later killed) by Hamas operatives in the West Bank. Israel launched a military operation to find the boys, arresting hundreds of Hamas members. Hamas militants in Gaza responded with rocket attacks. On July 2, a sixteen-year-old Palestinian from East Jerusalem was abducted near his home and burned to death by Israeli extremists in a revenge attack for the deaths of the Israeli teens. That death triggered yet more violent protests.

I was listening to the news as I cycled through Hyde Park on my way to St. Mary's when I heard that seven more Hamas militants had been killed by an Israeli airstrike. In retaliation, forty rockets were fired from Gaza into southern Israeli cities and towns. The following day, July 8, the Israel-Gaza war began, termed Operation Protective Edge by the Israelis. Their stated aim was to stop rocket fire from Gaza into Israel; Hamas's goal, conversely, was to bring international pressure to bear to lift Israel's blockade of the Gaza Strip, end the offensive, secure an independent third party to monitor and guarantee compliance with the ceasefire, secure the release of Palestinian prisoners, and overcome its political isolation. There was a lot at stake. But from a humanitarian point of view it was yet again a dire situation for the civilians on both sides.

Watching the news on television was soul-destroying. There was indiscriminate firing of rockets by armed groups in Gaza, and Israeli attacks on civilians in violation of international humanitarian principles. The intensity of the shelling, the number of deaths and injuries among the Palestinian civilian population and the extent of the infrastructural damage increased by the day.

A week after the war began, my cell phone rang. It was the International Committee of the Red Cross: would I go to Gaza City? The number of casualties was rising hourly and urgent surgical help was required. It was a no-brainer. A couple of phone calls to the managers at various hospitals confirmed that they were happy for me to leave immediately. That same day I was on a plane to Tel Aviv and from there on to East Jerusalem for a briefing.

The ICRC had been in Gaza since 1967, both protecting civilians and visiting people held in Israeli and Palestinian detention centers. It liaised with its sister organization the Palestinian Red Crescent, which ran Gaza's ambulances. In the 2008 war a team of ICRC surgeons had had considerable impact on the surgical healthcare facilities. My mission was the first time since then that a Red Cross surgeon had gone to give practical help.

I was briefed by the head of mission, who seemed unusually solicitous. He kept saying, "You do know this will be dangerous, very dangerous? We are expecting casualties from the ICRC delegation. Do you really want to go?" He was at pains to point out that they would do their best to ensure our safety, but could provide no guarantee. The situation was very hazardous.

I had already taken many risks in my life, and so far had emerged unscathed. In Bangui earlier that year I hadn't really thought about my personal safety at all; I'd go out for a walk after curfew, not bothered by the guns and the hostile stares. I'd seen it all before and had gotten away with it. This was just another gamble, and one worth taking. I wanted to be immersed in what was going on, and in a position to help people in direst need. This was my life; my heart was already racing in anticipation. Conflict work really was the only thing that made me feel alive.

We left East Jerusalem very early the following morning and reached the Erez Crossing at around 8:00 a.m., passing about thirty fully armored Israeli tanks on the way. As we had left our ICRC vehicle to be screened at the first checkpoint, it had struck me how underdressed we were, in our ordinary clothes with only a cotton ICRC tabard with the red cross emblazoned on the front and back to protect us—especially compared with the Israeli soldiers wearing body armor down to their knees and sturdy helmets, goggles, and masks. Their ground offensive was beginning that day. The situation was only going to get worse.

It took around two hours to pass through the checkpoint. To my surprise, among the people coming the other way, out of Gaza, I recognized someone I'd worked with in Haiti. She looked shell-shocked and told me that she had been there for only a week, but had found it absolutely terrible.

She wondered aloud, almost to herself, why on earth anybody would want to go there. She was distraught, almost hysterical. I was really worried for her.

I could see Gaza in the distance, with smoke billowing into the sky. And it wasn't long before I could see rockets coming toward us, too, until they were intercepted by the "iron dome"—Israel's air-defense system. It could destroy short-range rockets, artillery shells, and mortar fire from distances of up to forty-five miles. It was an amazing piece of equipment. A radar tracks the rocket as it is fired across the border, then advanced software predicts the rocket's trajectory. This information guides interceptor missiles fired from the ground to blow up the rockets. It was an extraordinary spectacle: I could see the rockets fired from Gaza followed by a line of white smoke and then, high above the Erez Crossing, they would suddenly disappear with a pop, blown into hundreds of pieces. But, of course, there was no such cover to protect Gaza.

Finally we were allowed to cross, and entered what resembled an airport lounge, fully air-conditioned against the searing heat outside. Again we went through the same checking of passports, who we were, why we were there, and so on, which took another two hours before we received permission to enter Gaza. This was an ordeal in itself. We had to drive through 200 meters of chicane, punctuated by enormous steel bollards rising up from the road before arriving at the next compound for more checks. At the last kiosk the checkpoint guard looked at us through his bulletproof screen and spoke into the loudspeaker: "Good luck, you'll need it, you're all crazy."

Once through the chicane, the last of the metal barriers opened and we could see the long, straight road toward Gaza City. As we edged nervously along it, we could see that the caged walkway on the left, which, we had been told, was usually full of people, was empty. We were going to do a kissing transfer, swapping rides with another vehicle whose passengers were leaving Gaza. We had to do this in the middle of the road, in full view, so that those watching from both the Gaza side and the Israeli side could see that security was not going to be compromised. We quickly changed vehicles and drove on down a road flanked by bombed-out houses. It was an eerie journey.

We headed for the ICRC headquarters in tense silence, until the driver received a message on his phone telling him to pull over and stop. There was about to be an airstrike. The shrieking of the fighter jets above us was deafening, then came the *boom-boom* of bombs being dropped. The raid ended after about twenty minutes, and we set off again.

On arrival in the center of Gaza City I was surprised to see a lot of people on the streets—I had been expecting everyone to be taking cover. We passed houses that had been bombed only minutes before, now ablaze and being attended to by firefighters. Several Palestinian Red Crescent ambulances with sirens wailing screeched past us on the way to pick up the wounded.

At the ICRC headquarters we had another briefing and I was introduced to the other members of the team. It was fairly small: I was the only surgeon, there was one emergency room physician who doubled as an anesthesiologist, several nurses, the head of security, a sanitation and water expert, and a fantastic lady named Kirrily Clarke, who was in charge of all the pre-hospital care carried out by the Palestinian Red Crescent. She liaised with both the Israeli authorities and Hamas, and had direct control of the Red Crescent ambulances. She was a Kiwi, and as tough as any All Black rugby player. Over the weeks that followed I watched in admiration as she stood her ground amid pressure from the warring parties.

I was embedded in the Shifa Hospital in the city, and quickly got down to work. Sometimes I operated on my own, supported by the ICRC team, but more often than not I worked with local surgeons. It was pure, hard-core war-trauma surgery, mostly dealing with the effects of bomb-blast injuries. There was a mass-casualty event most days, and it became quite normal to receive something like sixty or seventy patients in extremis, suffering the effects of an airstrike.

In academic terms, there are four categories of blast injuries. Category one is the effect of the initial shockwave that is generated when a bomb goes off. There is an instantaneous blast which creates an air shockwave that travels at supersonic speed and dissipates quickly over distance. When this shockwave goes through a human body it causes conditions such as shock lung, whereby the small blood vessels within the lung burst into one another and patients drown in their own blood. There may be no marks on the patient's body at all; all the damage is done inside.

Category two is the effect of shrapnel from the bomb itself or fragments of rubble from buildings damaged by the explosion. This is the kind of injury I had seen so often in Syria and elsewhere.

The original shockwave creates a vacuum. As it moves, the area behind rapidly fills up with fast-moving air, which gives rise to the so-called "blast wind." This is the category three effect. The blast wind can be so strong that it can lift a man up and throw him against a wall or other hard surface, and can sometimes cause traumatic amputation, literally taking off an arm or a leg. The other effects of the bomb, such as severe burns, or the effect of crush injuries due to falling debris, are category four.

Most of our patients were suffering in all four categories. To make things worse, infected flying debris and soil put them at risk of rapid death from septicemia. The treatment of blast injuries is extremely complex and challenging. We were treating up to sixty patients suffering from such injuries every day; the strain on the hospital and staff was enormous.

The hospital was almost always full to capacity, the emergency room abuzz with young doctors trying to resuscitate patients as they came through the door before quickly transferring them to one of the twelve operating rooms. If they were all busy, as was often the case, surgeons would operate on the floor or on gurneys. I frequently had to amputate the remains of an arm or a leg, sometimes in the most problematic areas, for example the junction between the chest and the shoulder, wearing a pair of rubber gloves and wielding a big pair of scissors and a few clips to clamp off the major blood vessels. These are not the sterile conditions in which such procedures should be conducted. There were so many casualties with so many significant injuries that each individual surgeon, no matter their grade or experience, just had to do their best to treat whoever was in front of them. There was no time to help other surgeons; as soon as your patient was dealt with, another would come along.

I was very impressed with the way they managed mass casualties. Often before going upstairs to surgery I would stand behind the senior surgeon, who was also the triage officer, and watch as he determined which cases needed immediate care and which could be put aside for a few hours. To be honest, though, the decisions were quite easy—almost everyone needed major surgery.

We worked through the day and into the night, and I regularly had to stay in the hospital because of the curfew. It was considered too dangerous to travel to or from the hospital during the night, and the ICRC's security mandate dictated that anyone in the hospital after a certain time must stay there. Similarly, anyone at the safe house during curfew could not return to the hospital in any circumstances.

Nights in the safe house were punctuated with noise from incoming rockets, which sometimes was relentless. And there did seem to be much more incoming fire than outgoing. It was frustrating, too, lying there knowing that any number of casualties were being transported to the hospitals, but we were immobilized by the security lockdown.

One night I was awoken at about one in the morning when my bed bounced off the floor. There had been an enormous explosion only meters away from the safe house. I lay in the dark wondering if we had been hit. On top of the house was a light that shone onto a red cross, to indicate that this was an ICRC residence, but it couldn't protect us from collateral damage, which was a regular occurrence.

More shells landed, the pounding getting closer and closer and the gap between explosions shortening. It seemed as if the entire neighborhood around us was being blown up. I leapt out of bed and threw open the metal shutter that protected the window. I had never seen anything like it. What looked like a heavy cloud overhead was lit up by searchlights. There were drones flying around, their flashing red lights indicating their location. Above the drones, fighter jets circled Gaza, firing indiscriminately into the city. Then, suddenly there was silence, swiftly followed by another intense battery of incoming artillery.

The safe house came alive, with the Dutch security manager running around shouting at everyone to get into the bunker. This was a concrete underground room, its entrance surrounded by sandbags. About fifteen of us sat through what sounded like the coming apocalypse. I had never before experienced such intense military action, not even in Iraq or Afghanistan.

Many of the people in the bunker were crying—not for themselves, but for the people who had to endure this absolute terror. The walls were creaking under the intense bombardment and even the dust shivered in the shockwaves.

I remember casting my eyes to the ceiling, thinking maybe my time was finally up. I really thought there was a very strong possibility that I might die there, and I would end up in the Gaza war cemetery, where some 3,217 British soldiers of the First World War are buried, many of whom died during the battle to take Gaza from the Ottomans in April 1917.

It wouldn't have been my first choice for a final resting place. I had already chosen the spot where I was going to be buried: with my parents in a family plot in the churchyard of the chapel of Bryn Moriah, about fifteen miles from Carmarthen on a small hill in the middle of nowhere. It is a windy place, surrounded by tall trees, and to be honest it's rather eerie. My mother and father lie between Mamgu and Datcu on one side, and, on the other, one of my cousins, who died in childbirth, and her baby. All the people in the row are related to each other and to me, and it seemed a fitting place for me to enter eternity.

But the Gaza war cemetery would be all right, I thought; even quite romantic. I was quite reconciled to the idea that I might die. But I did reflect on the fact that I had nobody to share that thought with, or talk about what was happening to me. It was hard to think straight, though, no matter how fatalistic I might have felt. What did it mean to carry on? How many lives saved was enough? Who was even keeping count? I had seen so much death, so many horrific sights; no one in their right mind could remain unaffected by it.

We sat there all night until the security manager allowed us to leave at about 7:30 in the morning, and I shuffled back to my room. But there was no way I could sleep; I wanted to go to the hospital and help deal with the night's carnage. As I got changed and packed my bag, a business card fell onto the floor. It carried the name of a young woman I had met just before coming to Gaza, at a Syria Relief fundraising event with Mounir. Her name was Eleanor, although people called her Elly. Her email address was on the card and, as I looked at it, I realized she was the one I wanted to talk to. I decided to email her. It seemed random enough that it wouldn't matter if she ignored my message, but I admit that, although we had only met for a few minutes, she had made my heart skip a beat. I quickly wrote a short email saying that I thought she was very nice, and that I just wanted her to know that. I still don't quite know why I did this, or what I thought would happen, but I pressed Send and went to work.

The hospital that morning was bedlam. All the operating rooms were busy with casualties and it was obvious that the staff had had no rest at all. They were exhausted, but there was still much work to be done. The gurneys in what was supposed to be the recovery bay were full of patients waiting for surgery. Some had already died; others were very sick and in need of urgent surgery.

As I walked around assessing the injuries and working out who should go to surgery, I came across a girl who looked about seven years old. She was lying on her own in the corner. She looked gray, and, to be honest, I thought she was dead. I checked her vital signs: her airway was clear but her breathing was very shallow. I checked for anemia by examining the inside of her lower eyelid—it was extremely pale, indicating that she had lost a lot of blood. I felt her wrist—the radial pulse was weak and thready and her blood pressure was low. There was nobody to ask what injuries she had, so I carefully removed the blanket that was covering her. She had obviously been involved in a blast injury and had a fragmentation wound to her left arm, which was bandaged. I had a quick look underneath the bandage and saw a massive defect at the front of the elbow. I examined her left radial artery and found no pulse. She must have had an arterial injury to that arm and required immediate revascularization. That wasn't all, her small bowel was hanging outside her body. This little girl was dying, and needed to go into surgery immediately.

I quickly went around the operating rooms to see which one I could use. In one they were just finishing an amputation, and I asked whether I could move in and operate on the child right away. Surprisingly, the outgoing surgeon said, "Be my guest." I think he had had enough. The Red Cross anesthesiologist was an excellent Italian fellow called Mauro Torre. He and I pushed the girl into the operating room ourselves and got her ready. I told the scrub nurse that I needed a vascular set as well as a general set of instruments. He ran off and picked up various items from other operating rooms to put together what I needed.

I watched her being put to sleep and then went into the corner of the OR to scrub up. As someone tied my surgical gown, I noticed a commotion outside; people were running to and fro in a panic. Suddenly, the door of the operating room flew open. It was the hospital security manager.

"We've got intel that says the hospital's going to be attacked by shelling in five minutes. Everyone out."

A few days earlier, I had been in another hospital in the center of Gaza when a missile had struck the hospital and gone straight through the intensive care unit, killing a number of patients and staff. The Israelis were apparently being told that some hospitals were harboring Hamas fighters, and targeted them as a result.

The scrub nurse looked very nervous as I plunged my left hand into one glove, which he was holding open, and my right hand into the other. The door of the operating room then swung open again; this time it was the ICRC security manager, who ordered us to leave immediately. Everybody else in the room began making a beeline for the door, joining the rest of the staff in the corridor heading out of the hospital as fast as they could.

The security manager began shouting at Mauro and me. "You have to go! Now! Right now!"

By this time, the little girl was asleep, and on the ventilator. She was a pitiful sight, her bowel hanging out of a hole in her abdominal wall and fragmentation wounds in her chest, arm, and abdomen. I looked at her blood pressure monitor, which read around 60 systolic. We would be leaving her in the OR uncovered, getting cold, and still bleeding internally. The time she had left to live could be counted in minutes, not hours, whether there was an airstrike or not.

By now everybody else had left the operating room. Even the security manager had gone to clear other rooms. Lots of things went through my mind. The most burning thought was that I could not leave this little girl to die on her own, having suffered the most extreme injuries. She was an innocent child and did not deserve such a fate. She had to be protected from this dreadful violence, not be part of it.

I was reminded of what had happened in Sarajevo all those years before. I had thought I might die then and had thought so during the shell attack on the safe house the previous evening. Maybe *this* was the moment it ended. And if it was, did I need to save myself? The answer, of course, was no.

I was on my own in the world, with no parents, no siblings, no wife, no children, and no dependents. In the grand scheme of things, it didn't much matter whether I lived or died; at least I would be doing something that I loved, and I might even save this girl in the process. I made a conscious decision to stay.

The patient was now fully anesthetized and the ventilator was working.

I turned to Mauro and said, "You can go, you don't need to stay."

"Are you staying?"

"I'm staying."

"Then I'll stay with you."

I brought my operating set to the table, and looked again at Mauro. Our eyes locked. It was a look that conveyed so much: part fear, part trepidation; a mixture of regret, respect, and farewell.

"You should go," I said again.

"No, David, I will stay with you."

He, too, was a veteran of many missions, also unmarried with no dependents. I suppose we had both been thinking the same thing.

So we stayed with the little girl, waiting for the bomb to drop or the missile to strike, or whatever it might be. I wondered what it would be like. But I calmly prepared the girl's abdomen with iodine, picked up the green drapes and clipped them into position. There was no rush; we took our time. I had a feeling of certain and impending doom, and flashed back to the checkpoint in the Congo, when I thought I was going to be shot in the neck. This time, though, it wasn't personal. I couldn't see the perpetrator of my death. I just knew it might be coming.

I made an incision the full length of her abdomen, from just below the breastbone to the pubic area. Inside was a large piece of shrapnel that had caused mayhem. It had entered in the right iliac fossa, around the hip bone, and the hole it had made had allowed the small bowel to escape. It had cut a hole in her bladder and in some parts of her small and large bowel and had also gone directly into the spleen, which was bleeding profusely. I strained to hear any sound of incoming rockets. Nothing. The hospital was silent. I looked at Mauro, who raised his eyebrows back at me.

The scrub nurse had left a lot of unopened swabs on the side and I asked Mauro to open them all up for me so I could pack her abdomen. The familiar process took my mind off the situation we were in, and by the time I'd removed her spleen and started mobilizing various parts of her bowel, Mauro told me twenty minutes had passed since we'd begun. Still no attack. There was nothing to do but carry on. We completed the operation, repairing the holes in her small bowel and colon, and making her abdomen look normal again. I then turned my attention to her left arm and repaired the artery damaged by another piece of shrapnel.

Two hours later, the operating floor was still deserted. We decided to wake her up in the operating room. As we were doing this, people started to drift back in, amazed to see us still there. Clearly, there was to be no attack.

I am not sure where the information had come from but I was told that it was a credible source—the ICRC was embedded with both sides—and that's why everybody had panicked and left. Nor do I know how many patients died in other operating rooms or what happened to them. I only knew that our little girl was alive and kept my fingers crossed that she would recover. I went to see her every day after that and got to know her family very well. Her name is Aysha and the photograph I have of me standing by her hospital bed, both of us smiling, says it all.

Unfortunately, though, I had ruffled a few feathers in the delegation, especially those of the security manager, who was livid. In the morning meeting a couple of days later, sitting around the table with all the other expats to discuss the previous day's events, I was told that I was being sent home. It was dressed up as a security issue: quite a few people were also going home because the situation outside was becoming so dangerous that the head of security felt it was only a matter of time before someone from the mission was killed.

Perhaps it had been irresponsible of Mauro and me to stay, but I felt in that moment that the girl's welfare took priority. It wasn't a logical decision, it was based purely on emotion—compassion for her and anger at the forces of war ranged against her. I was so sick of seeing badly injured children that I could not bear to see another one and stand idly by. Staying with her was a pointless act of defiance against the warmongers, but it would have been impossible to do otherwise. The nature of the risks I was taking had grown without my really noticing. I was prepared to die, and I would rather have died than lived with myself knowing I'd left her alone.

Being sent home felt like a punishment, though, and I was furious—and said as much, forcefully. As I was remonstrating with the security manager, I caught Kirrily's eye and she nodded to show she understood. I knew that she would speak to the head of mission on my behalf. Sure enough, the decision was quickly reversed and I stayed until the end of my mission three weeks later.

Toward the end of my time in Gaza I received an email from Lisa Yacoub, chief executive of a charity called Chain of Hope, which specializes in helping people around the world with severe cardiac problems. It had been set up by Lisa's father, the world-famous cardiac surgeon Sir Magdi Yacoub. She asked if I'd be able to help get permission for a three-year-old girl to be moved from Gaza to London. Before the war began, Chain of Hope had agreed to treat this child, Hala, who had a hole in the heart that could be repaired only in a major cardiac center.

Hala was born with a congenital heart defect. She lived in Beit Hanoun, a town in the northeast of Gaza, and had been earmarked for treatment by the Palestinian Children's Relief Fund, a wonderful charity that had teamed up with Chain of Hope. Her house was bombed during the war and she was living in dire circumstances in a UN school, cramped together in a corner of a room with her parents. There had been repeated attempts to get her evacuated, but to no avail. She had been severely traumatized by the bombing and had stopped speaking. By this point, she was unable to walk and was constantly attached to an oxygen cylinder for which no refill was easily available.

For Hala, time was running out. Her oxygen levels were so low that even the smallest movement turned her blue. She needed the operation as soon as possible. But there was no way of getting her out because of the intense bombing. That week, though, there would be a seventy-two-hour ceasefire; this was our chance. I wasn't due to leave Gaza for another week, but the opportunity to help Hala get out during the ceasefire was too good to miss. I went to the head of mission and asked if I could leave early and take her with me.

As I was a British Red Cross delegate and Chain of Hope was a British charity, I went through the British Red Cross to push the ICRC in Geneva to grant passage for Hala out of Gaza. To my amazement, the normal bureaucracy went out the window and the Red Cross issued an exit visa. The only thing we needed now was a medical visa allowing entry to the UK. Without this, Hala would not be able to leave, ceasefire or no ceasefire. It was therefore crucial that the British ambassador in Jordan granted permission, but it was almost the end of the week and the British Embassy in Amman was closed over the weekend.

I relayed this news to Lisa Yacoub, who went into action. The *Sun* newspaper was then running a campaign to try and save Hala. Journalists from the paper called the prime minister's office. I am not exactly sure what was discussed, but there may have been some frank exchanges about future headlines if David Cameron did not put pressure on the ambassador in Amman. Whatever was said, we were told that there was a strong possibility that the visa would be granted. All we had to do was get there.

On Friday, August 8, 2014, I took Hala, her mother Mahdeya, and a new oxygen cylinder in a Red Cross convoy to the Erez Crossing. After many hours negotiation we were in Israel. We swapped cars, and the three of us were driven to the Allenby Bridge, which crosses the River Jordan near the city of Jericho and connects the West Bank with Jordan.

For Hala and her mother, who had never left Gaza and had scant experience of officialdom, it must have been very frightening. I stayed with them throughout, although we were supposed to be separated. It took about four hours of arguing with the Israeli guards before we were finally let through. Mahdeya could not read or write, and my Arabic was terrible, but somehow we managed it. Once in Jordan, we were taken to a hospital, where Hala was kept overnight in intensive care. Her condition was very poor: her oxygen saturations, which normally should be around 99 percent, were just over 60.

During the night, the all-important medical visa was issued, and very early the next morning we headed to the airport to wait for our flight to London. It must have been very strange for Hala and her mother, who had been bombed out of their home, to be in the business lounge of a busy airport, of all places. Mahdeya was amazed when I produced cakes and sweets and sandwiches in abundance, all for free.

We boarded the plane, with Hala sitting between us. I had spoken to the flight attendant to ensure that there would be enough oxygen available for the whole flight. I hooked up the oxygen, put the nasal mask over Hala's face and the oxygen saturation probe on her little finger, and we settled ourselves in for the five-and-a-half-hour flight. A white-knuckled Mahdeya held on to the sides of her seat as we took off, frightened and anxious for both herself and her daughter.

Three hours into the flight, they both went off to the toilet, oxygen bottle in hand. They were gone a long time, around forty minutes, and I began to worry. What were they doing in there? Had something happened? Just as I was about to call the flight attendant, they came out. Hala had collapsed—her mother brought her back dangling in her arms unconscious. She had stopped breathing and was quite blue. I cleared everything off the seat and snatched the Ambu bag, a neat device for ventilating a patient, out of my first-aid kit. I had no way of knowing if her heart had stopped, but it certainly looked like it. I put the small oral airway into her mouth, which kept the space between her tongue and her windpipe open, and proceeded to hand-ventilate her. I shouted to the flight attendant but nobody was in earshot, and I couldn't find the call button among the array on the arm of the seat.

I went into full-on first-aid mode—luckily I had practiced the maneuver quite recently, on an obstetric and pediatric course a few months earlier. Three rescue breaths via the ventilator bag followed by two thumbs on the rib cage, pressing to stimulate a cardiac output. Do this thirty times and then give two rescue breaths. I turned the oxygen up to 100 percent. She was still floppy and there was no response. I began to panic. I shouted out "Help!" and the man in front hurried to find the flight attendant, who came at once. I told her that Hala was in cardiac arrest, most likely due to hypoxia, and that the captain needed to descend as rapidly as he could so that we could improve the oxygenation in the cabin. He responded immediately and suddenly Hala began to improve—she started to move and breathe and her dark-blue lips became lighter. The relief was overwhelming and I felt utterly elated. Believe it or not, this was the first time I had ever successfully performed cardiopulmonary resuscitation on my own.

The captain asked if we should divert to an airfield nearby, but we had only an hour left to go and I felt that with our diminishing altitude and maintaining as much oxygen flow as I could, we were altogether going to be OK. Fifteen or twenty minutes after this dreadful ordeal, Hala was sitting in her seat holding her teddy, her head resting on her mother's shoulder.

On landing we were met by Lisa and her team from Chain of Hope and we had a super-fast transit through Heathrow. I accompanied Hala in the ambulance down the M4 and through London, a speedy trip I am sure Lewis Hamilton would have been proud of. Even so, on arrival at Brompton Hospital, her oxygen saturation was only 40 percent. It was amazing that she was still alive.

A few days later, having been stabilized, she underwent open-heart surgery and a week after that she was transformed. A dying little girl had turned into the happiest, brightest little thing you could imagine. It was an absolute joy to see, and we held a party at the hospital to celebrate her recovery. It felt like a rebirth, and not only for Hala, but also for me, for there was another reason that occasion was so special: I took with me a plus one—the young woman I had emailed from Gaza.

I had emailed Elly again a few days before leaving Gaza. I told her I was coming back soon, and wondered if she'd like to meet me for a drink. We arranged to meet on the Saturday, the day I got back. But after the stress of the flight and dropping off Hala at the hospital, I began to regret the suggestion—I was shattered, and my mind was elsewhere, in a land full of bombs and bullets and damaged limbs. I texted to say maybe it wasn't such a good idea, but we could still meet if she wanted. She said she'd come, and we arranged to meet at the station at Imperial Wharf in Chelsea.

I had booked a table at a Thai restaurant nearby and arrived looking disheveled and feeling out of sorts. I saw her sitting on a concrete plinth outside the station. As I approached, I remembered how very beautiful she was. She stood up to greet me, and she was immediately warm and charming. I looked at her rather bemusedly, thinking how completely surreal the situation seemed. Here I was, not having washed in days, fresh from a journey in which I'd saved a child's life, looking like a wild man, thinking like a wild man, and somehow accompanying this lovely young woman to dinner.

In the restaurant we were surrounded by people laughing and chatting and having a good time, but I was finding difficulty in adapting to the fact that I wasn't somewhere where I might be blown up at any moment. The planes I heard flying overhead were not about to fire rockets at me but simply commercial airliners on their final approach to Heathrow. I looked around, trying to adjust, and couldn't quite believe there were people in the restaurant dressed in gorgeous summer clothes, seemingly without a care in the world.

I found it even more difficult to appreciate that I was now sitting opposite someone I'd only emailed because I'd thought that I was going to die. It seemed an inauspicious way to begin whatever this was, or might become. I had had many disastrous relationships in the past, some lasting longer than others, but they had all fallen by the wayside. I had always longed for a partner, maybe even a family, but simply had not met the right person. I assumed, too, that there was no one who could possibly want me. I still harbored a sliver of hope, though; maybe this would be the final roll of the dice.

But that evening there was a complete disconnect between my heart and my head. I looked at Elly and could not get over how ridiculous it was that this charming woman was even sitting opposite me. I began to mumble and fumble for amusing conversation, but the words would not come. I was mesmerized by her. How could this be? It was hopeless. But she was so kind, so comforting and understanding. I think she saw I was struggling and within a few minutes told me that if I felt uncomfortable then it was no problem for her to go, we could arrange to meet another time if I wanted.

I sipped my first glass of red wine and decided to stay. As the evening went on it became much easier, and by the end of the meal I was in love. It's as simple as that. I knew that this was the woman I had been waiting for all of my life. It was as if Elly had rewired my brain, and by the end of the evening we were laughing and joking together and I felt I had known her all my life. Walking by the river on that hot August night, watching the lights shimmer on the Thames, I leaned over and held her hand and thought my heart might burst.

After that first date she had to go abroad on a business trip, and I went to a conference in Washington. But when we were both back in London we met up again and for the next two weeks were inseparable. I even met her parents, hoping beyond hope that they liked me, because by that time there was nothing either of us could have done to stop what had blossomed between us.

But separation loomed: I was due to fulfill my promise to Mounir and Ammar and the other surgeons and go back to Aleppo. I had three weeks to tie up my commitments at Chelsea and Westminster and at St. Mary's, after which I would be away for the next six.

A few days before I left for Syria, Elly had another business trip herself. We were both in tears as I dropped her off at Heathrow. It seemed nothing short of miraculous that this person had come into my life. I had felt adrift, swimming alone far out at sea, in increasingly dangerous waters, and it was as if someone had thrown me a lifeline. As she left for the departure gate, I promised her that I would be back. "I'll see you soon," I said. But part of me didn't believe that. Part of me thought that this would be the last time I would see her. I was quite certain the mission to Syria would be my last. Not because I no longer wanted to volunteer, but because I was not sure I would survive.

- 11 -
THE RAZOR'S EDGE

The plan was much the same as in 2013: a week at the hospital at Bab al-Hawa, in the north, then on to Aleppo for five weeks. This time, though, we would have a camera crew in tow—Channel 4 was making a documentary about emergency healthcare on the front lines in Syria. The producer would fly out with us and train up a local Syrian camera crew. But first I was filmed packing my gas mask and other surgical equipment in my flat before we set out.

We met Ammar in Istanbul and the three of us then flew to Hatay, the closest airport to the Turkey-Syria border. I hadn't realized quite how much equipment the producer was bringing with him until we went through customs, where he was stopped. He told them we were making a documentary about birdwatching in Turkey, but it must have been patently obvious what we were doing—how on earth we got through customs, I'll never know.

We loaded up the car that had been sent for us and got around half a mile from the airport before we were intercepted by three police cars. We were all forced out of the car and every document and every box of camera gear was scrutinized. We stuck to the same story. After an hour or so they sent us on our way, with a stark warning that if it didn't check out, we would be locked up.

We stopped briefly in Reyhanlı, before Ammar and I were driven to the border crossing and then on to Bab al-Hawa. The producer stayed in Reyhanlı to teach and train the cameramen who were going to follow us. Meeting the team at the hospital, some of whom had been there the previous year, was a joy. It didn't take long before there were plenty of patients lining up to see us. Most had been injured by bullets or fragments and had festering wounds that needed covering. There were no hospital beds for long-term care, so patients were usually discharged quickly. Their dressings were rarely changed under sterile conditions, so the wounds had become infected, and some of them turned into permanently open wounds, posing a significant risk to the patient. Many patients who had both orthopedic and soft-tissue injuries were discharged with their external fixators still in place, and because nobody knew how to cover the bone, the bone was left exposed, too.

Soon enough around half the people in the outpatients' department that had been set up for me had this type of injury. The rest were those with severe scarring from burns on their bodies, sometimes with terrible burn contractures that contorted their faces. Over the last twenty years I had become a fairly competent amateur plastic surgeon, but in war zones the aesthetic bar is somewhat lower than, say, Beverly Hills. I am able to do most of the rudimentary work required, but there was a lot to do.

I was delighted to see that Bab al-Hawa, previously a Customs and Excise building, had become a fully functioning hospital with four operating rooms. The bed capacity had also increased, to around forty, and it had become a district general hospital. None of this could have happened without the constant help and support of the charities working around the clock to provide financial support to convert the building and pay the staff.

I had been given an operating room with an anesthesiologist and scrub staff twenty-four hours a day for my elective work, but the hospital was still receiving patients with fresh injuries. As well as the usual gunshot wounds and fragmentation injuries from airstrikes, we saw the devastating effects of the regime's new weapon of choice: barrel bombs. Helicopters took off from Syrian regime bases carrying large steel drums packed with 1,100 pounds of TNT, and a detonator at the base. The helicopters hovered at around 3,000 feet over their targets, often civilian areas and, increasingly, hospitals, then dropped the bombs. I had not seen the horrific consequences of a barrel bomb before, but that would soon change.

While I was in Bab al-Hawa I was delighted to be joined by two of my great friends from the previous trip: Abdulaziz, now working in Turkey, but regularly crossing the border to perform lifesaving surgery in Aleppo, and my young plastic surgeon friend Abu Waseem.

Ammar, Abu Waseem, and I operated almost eighteen hours a day during that first week at Bab al-Hawa. Soon, though, it was time to move on to Aleppo. Another of our friends and colleagues, the urologist Abu

Mohammadain, met us at the hospital and we discussed the next leg of the journey. Castello Road was still the only way in and out of the city, but it was even more perilous now. It was surrounded on all sides by regime forces. Only a narrow channel remained open. Abdulaziz was careful to warn us how dangerous and difficult it was.

As on my last mission, it helped to rationalize things if I knew more about what was going on. The friction I had seen beginning in 2013 had reached a fairly inevitable conclusion, with significant clashes between ISIS and the Free Syrian Army, many of whose members had been subjected to horrendous torture in the same police station that Ammar and I had been inadvisably driven past. The FSA's patience ran out and there was intense fighting between them and ISIS, with around 2,500 fighters from each side killed. Most of the ISIS fighters who survived then moved to bolster their occupation of a large area around Raqqa.

Of course, the biggest beneficiary of this sideshow was Assad's regime. The government intensified its campaign of barrel-bombing Aleppo. This forced many residents to flee to the countryside, where the shelling was less intense. Abdulaziz told me that during February and March around seven hundred barrel bombs had been dropped, killing about 1,000 people and wounding another 4,000.

In June 2014 ISIS had declared its caliphate, stretching from northern Syria to western Iraq. There was intense fighting along a line from Aleppo to Turkey between the rebels and ISIS, who were only around twenty miles away from the city but were being kept at bay by the Free Syrian Army. The gap along Castello Road seemed to be closing in, with the Syrian military only a mile or two away on either side, constantly pounding the road.

"Do you really want to go in, David?" Abdulaziz asked.

Abu Waseem said he was going back anyway; he and Abu Mohammadain were leaving the next day. Ammar and I sat and talked for a while. He was Syrian, too, and wanted to go with them. So did I. They were my friends and colleagues and I didn't want to see them leave without me; more importantly, I wanted to help the people of Aleppo again. The deal was struck: we would leave the following morning at six.

As usual, we went in two cars. Ammar and I were in the second, driven by a man who said he was there to protect us. We laughed—he certainly looked the part. He was fully geared-up with body armor, a helmet, and a sidearm, while we only had a few cardboard boxes in the back of the car to protect us if we were shot at. Ammar joked that we'd use the driver as our human shield, like standing behind someone wearing a lead apron in a radiology department. However, there were a few AK-47s on the front seat. We supposed he would give them to us if necessary, and train us how to use them on the fly. As before, the journey down took three to four hours. There were fewer checkpoints this time, as ISIS had been forced back, but instead we had the threat from the regime, which was much closer.

Once we reached Castello Road we could see dozens of cars and trucks on the side of the road, some completely destroyed and others bearing the scars of rocket attacks. Some of them must have driven off the road at high speed to get away from the encircling jets, as there were still tire marks and track marks in the sand coming to an abrupt halt where the driver and occupants had been killed—I was certain their bodies must still be inside the wreckage of their vehicles. It was clearly far too dangerous for anybody to go and pick them up. It was like something out of a Mad Max movie.

This stretch of the journey took forty-five minutes—forty-five minutes of acute anxiety. We were very exposed, and as a result drove very fast. We finally reached the outskirts of Aleppo and the difference from the previous year was immediately visible. Where in 2013 there had been shops, markets, and people, now there was only destruction on an industrial scale. And because of the general exodus to the countryside, there were also far fewer people on the streets.

As before we went first to M10. Here another difference became apparent: to enter the hospital we now walked down a ramp—the hospital's main rooms had all been moved underground. M10 had been targeted by the regime in recent months and the infrastructure of the hospital I had worked in the previous year had been totally destroyed. Abu Mohammadain showed me the effects of the bombardment on the intensive care unit upstairs. The beds were still there, but the walls had gone, and there was dust and debris strewn across the floor. Perched above a collapsed bookshelf was a little red toy tractor that I had spotted the year before. It seemed to be the only thing to have survived the intensity of the attack. Abu Mohammadain told me that all six patients in the intensive care unit had died that day, as did many patients on the other wards upstairs that were now also in ruins.

But they had done the most amazing job—they had built a fully functional hospital in the basement. Traveling to and from the hospital was so dangerous that the staff now all lived together in a dedicated domestic area. There were two operating rooms, with good ventilation, lighting, and anesthesiology equipment. There was a new intensive care unit with six beds, all with their own ventilators, and an emergency room where patients would arrive after their journey down the ramp.

After a quick meal at M10 we drove to M1. Abu Hozaifa, one of the young surgeons I had trained in vascular surgery, had now become the vascular surgeon for the whole of Aleppo at only twenty-seven—he had cases being transferred to him from all over the city. Within half an hour of arriving we were back in the operating room together, where I assisted him with a tricky fragmentation injury to a patient's thigh. I was amazed by his transformation from a rather junior surgeon to a really experienced vascular surgeon in just twelve months.

That evening, we all sat and talked upstairs in the dining room. There were two new general surgeons who I was yet to meet, but the rest of the team was the same apart from a couple of junior surgeons who had left. We were a family again, and I was enormously proud to be back.

I could not help noticing, though, that their demeanor was different. They looked drained, hollow. They were under constant barrage from barrel bombs and also from the jets that shot anything that moved with rockets and machine guns. Simply getting around the city had become exceptionally dangerous, more so in the last few months than ever before. The chance of being killed simply moving from one hospital to another was something like one in four. The previous year there had been around 2 million people living in Aleppo, now it was down to 350,000—the ones who'd stayed were too ill to leave, or too stubborn—or, of course, too poor. One of the new doctors helpfully told me my chances of leaving the city alive were fifty-fifty.

As we sat there, we could hear helicopters above our heads. I went over to the blown-out window and was told to be careful: no one knew where the bombs were going to fall; you had to track the low hum of the helicopters and quickly head to the bomb shelter if the engine noise got louder. Sometimes the helicopters would drop their barrel bombs from as high as 10,000 feet, and at that altitude you could not hear them at all. The first you'd know of it was the explosion.

I spent a restless night wondering what was going to happen over the next few weeks. The atmosphere in the hospitals and among my colleagues was quite different: tense, charged. It felt altogether edgier and more dangerous than my previous trip, and I wondered once again whether I had bitten off more than I could chew.

I was woken the next morning by the sound of explosions. Some of the blasts were clearly far away, but one was particularly close, and the whole hospital shook. Ammar and I got up, changed into our surgical scrubs and went down to the operating rooms. We could hear the sirens of approaching ambulances and soon the casualties arrived in the emergency room. They were all completely covered in white dust, as if they had been rolling in flour. One man sitting in a corner had streaks of blood etched into the creases of his skin. Three or four patients were lying on gurneys and the dust on them was so thick it was impossible to tell which way they were facing.

This was a pernicious side effect of the barrel bombs. Most of Aleppo's major buildings were made of concrete, and when struck by the bomb they exploded into clouds of toxic dust, covering everyone inside or anywhere nearby. I couldn't tell whether one of these patients was a man or a woman, or even which side was facing up. There must have been half an inch of dust all over their head. I was given a wet rag, which turned out to be the most useful medical implement to carry, because it allowed you to wash the dust away and see which way the face was turned. I gradually revealed a woman. I opened her mouth only to find it was full of concrete dust. And, of course, she was dead.

I went over to the other patients to help. The same thick dust was washed off a young child, who had a terrible fragmentation injury to his leg—he'd lost the lower part of one leg and the middle part of his thigh. He had obviously also lost a lot of blood, so I applied a tourniquet and called an anesthesiologist to get him into surgery as quickly as we could. One of the new surgeons looked decidedly unimpressed, so I turned to Ammar and asked him to help me. We spent about three hours operating on the boy, but unfortunately he had inhaled too much dust and died a few hours later.

Shortly afterward I found the new surgeon, who told me that in his view the whole exercise was completely pointless—everyone he had operated on who'd been covered in dust had subsequently died. He didn't exactly say, "Don't bother," but he was increasingly convinced that anyone who came in after a barrel-bomb attack would die. He thought I'd arrived fresh from the outside world with little understanding of what it was now like in Aleppo—and it was certainly a stark contrast to 2013. Then, almost all our work had been on gunshot wounds and we had saved a lot of lives—in some weeks every patient who came to us was saved. It was obvious this doctor was very depressed and had become extremely cynical. Tensions were high and the constant daily barrage was taking a significant toll on the mental health of all the hospital staff.

Day after day we saw entire families brought in, their homes destroyed by barrel bombs. But it was only very rarely that the father was with them—the men were either trying to find food or involved in the fighting. Most of the children we saw were under ten. Some were dead on arrival, covered in dust but with no other marks on them: they had either died from the effects of the shockwave or had suffocated from inhaling pulverized concrete. Others had fragmentation injuries from the bombs or from red-hot flying debris. We spent hours in the operating room trying to patch people up and to relieve the suffering as best we could.

Mercifully, for a few days in the middle of this mission it went quiet, with no air attacks and no barrel bombs. Abu Mohammadain reminisced about how beautiful Aleppo had been before the war, and how all religions and creeds had existed in harmony. We began speaking about religion and God, and I asked him if he knew of any Christian churches still open. There was one, apparently, in the old city.

While I'm not religious in terms of going to church every week, I do believe there is a God, and have called on his help on occasion, as I've already mentioned. Over the past few weeks, I had seen a lot of death; I felt closer to God than I had for a long time and had a powerful urge to pray. I knew also that Elly went to the church near her office at lunchtime whenever she could and was praying for me there.

Ammar and I and a few others went with Abu Mohammadain in his beat-up car to M2, another trauma hospital that was close to the front line. There, we were met by a paramedic who knew the area well and had agreed to escort us to the church. We headed out via some backstreets and ended up in the old city. Where the buildings were still standing, it was easy to see how beautiful Aleppo had once been. We walked around the souk, where all the shops were now deserted and abandoned. Our guide then took us into a fountain-filled courtyard. Miraculously, he was able to turn them on, and cascades of water shot into the air, hitting the sunlight and making a rainbow. Amid all the horrors of the war, it was a breathtaking sight.

We went down some steps into a bathhouse, its blue marble mosaic beckoning the ghosts of past bathers, and then continued past wooden houses whose upper stories hung over the narrow streets, weaving our way toward the great Umayyad Mosque. Built at the beginning of the eighth century, it was supposedly home to the remains of Zachariah, the father of John the Baptist. Its minaret had been completed in 1090 and must have been very beautiful, but it had been almost totally demolished by the bombing. The mosque's past glory was difficult to imagine now, so ruined was it. There were holes in the walls filled with rubber tubes which acted as gun turrets. It was painful to see a place of such architectural and spiritual beauty treated so disrespectfully.

We finally made it to an open space. Only a wall now separated us from territory held by the Syrian regime. I looked through a gap in the wall and saw a Syrian government flag. We were as close to the front line as you could get. I asked our guide how it was that parts of the old city were still relatively well-preserved and was told that it was because this front-line wall was so close to areas occupied by the regime; they did not want to bomb their own side by mistake.

We wandered on, stopping at another open area that had once been a playground. It was deserted now, and silent apart from the sound of a battered swing creaking in the wind. The playground had been converted into a graveyard and our guide went over to one of the plots, where he stood quietly for a few minutes. His two sisters and his mother were buried there.

Finally, we arrived at our destination, the Mar Elias nursing home for the elderly. It was just off a small cobbled street and marked by a swinging sign pointing to a door. Opening this door was like passing into the Garden of Eden, such was the contrast with the mayhem and destruction outside. A statue stood in the center of a lushly planted courtyard. The priest I had come to see greeted us with a warm smile. Michel Abou Yousef clasped my hand in both of his, and beckoned us over to a table laid with china cups and plates. As Ammar translated, he told me his story.

The Mar Elias housed a Catholic chapel within its walls, where Michel had worked for many years. He had moved into the home after his house had been blown up, looking after the elderly residents who had stayed behind either by choice or necessity. Every day he would go to the market to buy food for the residents and cook it for them. He felt fairly safe there, as it was so close to the wall that divided east and west Aleppo.

As we were talking, some of the residents emerged from their rooms to see what was going on. We were soon surrounded by the old and infirm, but what struck me was how calm and happy they all seemed. Perhaps they had become oblivious to the noise of gunfire and the occasional thud of a bomb being dropped. These had become such a feature of the city's soundtrack that nobody took any notice.

Michel looked tired and drawn, much older than his fifty-three years. He had been ordained as a priest many years ago and was confident that God would help them in the end. He asked me my religion. A Protestant, I told him, Church of England, in fact. Smiling, he said we were all children of God. He suggested we could pray together, and asked if I would like him to bless me in his little chapel. I said it would be a great honor. With this, he went off for about fifteen minutes before reappearing in the robes of an ordained Catholic priest.

We opened the doors of the little chapel. Inside was an altar with a couple of candles and a picture of Christ above it. He beckoned me to kneel with him in front of the altar and said a few words. I did not understand the precise meaning of what he was saying, but I could hear the compassion in his voice. Before I knew what was happening tears were rolling down my face. The carapace I had built up over the past few weeks—the past few decades—was in danger of cracking.

Michel disappeared for a moment, returning with a small cup, which he filled with wine. He placed a wafer on my tongue and offered me the cup. He then placed his hand on my head and prayed. For the second time in my life I felt this contact not as something physical but as a spiritual connection; it did not feel like a man's hand but something much more powerful and profound, radiating energy. An electric shiver ran through me, filling me with love. The first time I had experienced this had been only a few weeks before, when I was at dinner with my great friend Richard Smith, a consultant gynecologist. Richard is a man of great faith and has a small consecrated chapel in his house. He prayed for me before I went to Syria. When Richard had placed his hand on my head, it had also been an intensely spiritual moment. The emotion I felt then—and now, in Aleppo—was all-consuming.

Michel left me to compose myself and when I went back outside I found him sitting with Ammar, Abu Mohammadain, and our guide, surrounded by elderly residents of the home, all of whom clearly loved him very much.

It encapsulates everything about Syria's tragedy that this moment of grace should have an unhappy ending. Within days, the man who had guided us so generously through the old city was killed in an airstrike. And six months later Michel himself was killed, during a barrel-bomb attack while shopping for food for his flock. What happened to the people he was caring for, God only knows.

On the short journey back to M1, we were stopped at an armed checkpoint. We weren't sure who the guards at the checkpoint were, and Abu Mohammadain spent quite some time telling them we were doctors simply going from one hospital to another. We were dressed in our surgical scrubs to prove the point. Everyone knew Abu Mohammadain and he knew everyone, so the fact that they claimed not to recognize him made things a little tense. He was taken into the guards' bombed-out shelter to provide further details, but the rest of us were allowed to carry on and decided to walk. It was less than a mile to M1.

Back in east Aleppo, the ruined streets were deserted. No one walked anywhere if they didn't have to; it was simply too dangerous. We passed a school that had been bombed. It must have been at least four or five stories high, but was now flattened. On the ground floor you could still see child-sized desks and chairs poking out from the rubble. The smell of death seemed more concentrated here than elsewhere; there must have been children in the building when the bomb fell.

We were hurrying now, anxious to be home. Suddenly, the unearthly calm was shattered by the arrival of a Syrian fighter jet overhead. We were out in the open and the pilot had obviously seen us. He turned in a hard circle to come around again. The four of us froze. Ammar began shouting for us to take cover, but there was nowhere to take cover apart from a wall some distance away. We ran toward it and crouched down as the plane came around once more, waiting for the moment to strike. As I stood next to Ammar, I was convinced that this would now be the end. I could see the jet coming directly toward us. The noise of the engines became deafening, but even that was then drowned out by the blast of the rockets hitting the buildings around us. I felt the shockwave, there was a high-pitched whine, and then nothing. We were on the ground huddled together. The intensity of my emotions were so high that I was unsure whether I was alive or dead.

As quickly as it had come, the jet disappeared. We were badly shaken, but otherwise unhurt. Finally back at the sanctuary of M1, we told colleagues what had happened. They shrugged their shoulders—for them, this kind of thing was a daily occurrence. The jet, or another from its squadron, had obviously continued its deadly work. It wasn't long before we heard there were heavy casualties at M10. Abu Mohammadain was back with us following his short detention, and we bundled into his car.

There were several ambulances outside M10 when we arrived. The situation inside was desperate. About forty people had been injured by rocket strikes or barrel bombs. Along one side of the emergency room there were about fourteen or fifteen people who were clearly already dead; some were in a terrible state, with limbs missing. The rest of the patients were being triaged by the young nurses while relatives of the wounded put up drips.

The surgeons had already begun operating and Ammar and I went to help. Many of the patients had gaping wounds at their extremities where limbs had been taken off by the blast. These required immediate surgery to staunch the hemorrhage and cut away as much of the damaged muscle and skin as quickly as possible before packing the wounds with gauze. Other patients had abdominal injuries in need of basic damage control—ligating the bowel, packing the abdomen with gauzes, and closing the skin rapidly.

At around three o'clock that afternoon, we heard a colossal bang nearby. Twenty minutes later yet another group of casualties arrived. I decided to document what was happening on my iPhone and stood at the entrance of the emergency room filming. What I saw will stay with me for the rest of my life.

A family of seven children came in with their mother. The mother had died and joined the bodies placed near the wall. The first child was just a toddler, and had lost both her feet. Her brother on the next gurney was about seven—he had a massive pelvic injury with parts of his small bowel coming through a large hole just above the hip bone. Another boy, about the same age, had blood streaming from his face and head but was obviously not seriously injured. But he was terribly traumatized, crying and shouting.

What happened next was so dreadful that I still have nightmares about it and hesitate to describe it here. Another little boy, about five years old, was brought in, face down on the gurney. Both his buttocks and the backs of his thighs had been completely blown off, and there were bits of what appeared to be cobwebs of tissue and dust and fragments of wire coming out of his wounds.

The nurses turned him onto his back. He was still alive, but was completely silent as he gazed around the room. On his face and hair were blobs of gray-white tissue I could not identify. One of the nurses pulled his hair back from his face and started to comb it gently with her fingers. That was all we could do for him; we had run out of morphine. A few minutes later another child was brought in, his sister. Half of her head and brain were missing. Some of what was missing was now splattered across her brother's face. They must have been playing together when the barrel bomb blew up their house and destroyed their lives.

I have seen many dreadful sights and had often thought I was inured to suffering. This, though, was beyond words. I felt sick—physically and emotionally. I was genuinely shocked by the devastation wrought on these innocent children.

We turned the little girl on her side to see her face. Like her brother, she was beautiful, with curly blonde hair. Her brother died after about twenty minutes, and we spent the rest of the day operating on his surviving siblings.

We finished at around ten o'clock that night, exhausted and numbed from the day's events.

After a disturbed night's sleep I woke to the inevitable sound of sirens. A patient was brought into the emergency room with a single fragmentation wound. The fragment had taken out the femoral artery in the left groin and he had bled so profusely that he was in cardiac arrest. One doctor was pressing on his groin trying to stem the hemorrhage while another performed CPR by rhythmically pressing on his chest. An anesthesiologist had already intubated and was ventilating him.

The body normally contains about five liters of blood. If a peripheral artery is cut then the patient will lose a lot of it. Because the cardiac output from the left ventricle is around five liters per minute, significant arterial damage can cause the entire blood volume to be lost in a very short period of time. The brain needs oxygen, which is delivered via the blood, and coma rapidly ensues if it does not get enough. In this situation the heart has very little blood left in it, so cardiac massage has almost no benefit. A quick decision has to be made about whether to attempt to save the patient or let them die. Time is literally of the essence: if the brain is starved of oxygen for longer than three or four minutes it will be irreversibly damaged, while lack of blood in the coronary arteries will cause segments of the heart to die, leading to a massive heart attack.

The procedure that's required is called a resuscitative thoracotomy. The left side of the chest is opened from the sternum through the ribs below the nipple as far down as possible. Having divided all the intercostal muscles, a rib-spreader is used to expose the lungs and the heart. Once the pericardium—the thick lining around the heart—is opened then both hands can be placed around the heart to perform *internal* cardiac massage. This way you can feel how much blood there is in the heart. If the heart feels empty, then the next maneuver is to place a clamp on the distal thoracic aorta, which is below the heart. This cuts off all the circulation to the rest of the body, apart from the heart itself and the head and arms. By pouring in blood through a central line in the neck, the heart and brain can be perfused with oxygenated blood.

Any decision to perform this procedure is dependent on the fact that external cardiac massage has been performed for only a few minutes. The chances of survival deteriorate with every passing second—the standard teaching is no more than fifteen minutes of external cardiac massage and ventilation, but in the real world it is often much less than this.

Our patient came in having had external cardiac massage for just two or three minutes. An immediate decision was needed about whether to operate. Leaving him meant that he would die; going ahead with an operation would give him a very slim chance of survival, but would probably also use up a lot of our blood, and there wasn't that much left in the bank.

On average, to fix someone with a penetrating injury to an artery that has led to external cardiac massage requires around twenty-five units of blood—and, obviously, these must be units of the right type. We had ten units of blood in total, never mind the correct type for this patient. At least one person present, the cynical Syrian surgeon, made it clear he thought operating would be futile and we should let him die. But we had all seen so much misery and death by now, and here was a barrel-bomb victim who *might* survive. His wife and child had also been brought in following the barrel-bomb attack, with minor injuries. We decided to rush him into surgery and do all we could to save him.

Someone was dispatched to try to locate some more blood from other hospitals while we wheeled the patient into the OR and began the thoracotomy. The operation went well and within half an hour or so his heart was beating nicely and he had good pupillary reflex, indicating that the brain was getting enough oxygen. Maybe we had caught him in time; maybe this would be a rare success. We took him to the intensive care unit, but as soon as we had done so we were called to another hospital to treat more casualties.

We returned to M1 about ten hours later. Our patient's leg was now the major cause of concern—one of the shunts we had been put in was obviously blocked, and the leg had had no circulation for several hours. That this had not been noticed by the nursing staff is unsurprising in such a chaotic situation. The worst of it, though, was that the man had by this point been given around forty units of blood; there was no blood left in Aleppo for anybody else. We slowly watched him die, knowing that if he had been anywhere else in the world he would probably have survived. Had we done the right thing in trying to save him, or should we have let him die earlier? My world-weary colleague looked at me as if to say, "I told you so."

What was already an exceptionally difficult mission then became even more fraught. Toward the end of September 2014 the Americans had launched their first airstrike on ISIS in Syria, and there was talk that other coalition countries had been involved too, including the United Kingdom. Over breakfast, one of the surgeons at M1 said that the strikes had killed Syrian civilians, not just ISIS fighters. He looked at me as if it was my fault and said, "The West are now killing us."

This exchange made me feel very uneasy, and I ducked out of breakfast as soon as I could. The doctor had always been a friend, and we had worked closely together on many cases both this year and the year before. But now he seemed to see me differently; I was an emissary of "the West."

The mission in 2013 had been hard, but ultimately successful and rewarding. In 2014 it was completely different. The danger, the pressure, the frustration, the wretched reality of life in Aleppo all compounded one another. We were walking on a razor's edge. Everyone was tired and stressed and tensions ran high. Arguments between close friends became more and more common, and although we all tried to remain stoical it was an uphill struggle.

Ammar told me that everyone, especially the Free Syrian Army, was increasingly disgruntled by the lack of support from the West. The army needed weapons, and the people needed money and food. Neither was forthcoming, and yet ISIS and other extremist groups who claimed to be against the Assad regime seemed to have a lot of money. Some were tempted to join them, if only to feed their families, and FSA numbers began to dwindle in the face of these temptations—and the effort of fighting the regime.

I tried to keep myself sane by occupying myself with the patients, even though about 80 percent of those who came in after a barrel-bomb attack died. I'd had minimal contact with Elly, for security reasons, but I thought about her often. What had we begun, and where might it lead? It was impossible to imagine, so remote did our relationship seem now. Slowly I became as miserable and cynical as the surgeon I'd met at the start of the mission.

In one respect I was shielded both from the outside world and from what was happening in Syria around me. I did, though, want to find out the situation concerning the airstrikes, and early one morning while everyone was asleep I found myself reading the BBC News website. It wasn't just the airstrikes that were bothering me, it was the fact that Westerners were being kidnapped and beheaded by ISIS not that far from where I was.

I read about James Foley, an American freelance journalist kidnapped in the north of Syria on his way to Turkey in November 2012—around the time I was working for MSF in Atmeh. He was beheaded in or around Raqqa in August 2014, apparently in retaliation for US-led airstrikes against the Islamic State in Iraq. His murderer was dubbed "Jihadi John," on account of his London accent, and was later identified as Mohammed Emwazi, a Kuwaiti-born jihadist who had moved to the UK with his family when he was six. Emwazi threatened that a second American would be killed if the airstrikes did not stop. He was true to his word. Steven Sotloff, a *Time* magazine journalist, had been kidnapped by ISIS in Aleppo when I was there in 2013. He was beheaded in early September 2014, in response to further American airstrikes in Iraq.

Just over the border from Turkey in Atmeh, a British aid worker named David Haines had been abducted in March 2013. He was beheaded in mid-September 2014. After the video of the beheading was broadcast, the executioner was shown with another British aid worker, Alan Henning, saying, "If you, [David] Cameron, insist on fighting the Islamic State then you, like your master Obama, will have the blood of your people on your hands." Henning was a forty-seven-year-old taxi-driver from Salford who had been kidnapped at one of the checkpoints on the way to Aleppo while driving an aid-organization ambulance. In late 2013 he had crossed from Turkey and was captured only half an hour's drive into Syria. He was still being held captive, probably less than an hour's drive from where I was.

I became extremely nervous after David Haines's execution, and every morning I obsessively tried to access the Internet, watching for news of Alan Henning. I would sit on the mattress in our small room, turn the brightness down on my computer so that I didn't disturb anyone, and follow the desperate situation that was unfolding.

I don't think I had realized the gravity of being a Westerner so deep inside Syria, perhaps the only free Westerner in the whole country at that time. I felt safe enough with my colleagues, and knew that Ammar and Abu Mohammadain would make sure nothing happened to me. I kept it to myself, but I was slowly heading down a rabbit hole. I had a near-constant pain in the middle of my chest, which I could ignore only when I was immersed in an operation. As well as the beheadings and the risk of kidnap and execution, I could not stop thinking about the previous year's run-ins—the ISIS invasion of the operating room and the poor man who'd been pulled off the ward and beheaded in the street.

One morning in early October someone came in and said, "Oh, Henning's been killed, do you want to see?" And like an idiot, I did see, and watched the terrible footage of his execution. I think it was this that tipped me over the edge. This awful thing had happened to another Brit, a volunteer just like me, not very far away. Hundreds of people in Aleppo knew who I was, and that I was there. Everybody had a cell phone—just one call, and that would have been it for me.

Abu Waseem had relatives in a village near Raqqa and often took the bus to visit them. He made sure that his cell phone was completely empty of content—he had seen people pulled off the bus at the numerous ISIS checkpoints along the way because they had something on their phone that the jihadists took exception to. He'd even known people who were strict in their religious adherence who had been abducted in this fashion and never seen again. It could happen to anyone. As a Westerner I would be a prized scalp; my status as a doctor offered no protection whatsoever.

I began to feel very isolated and tried to keep as low a profile as possible, even in the hospitals—maintaining a neutral, pleasant demeanor and not saying too much. It was very easy to become paranoid if somebody looked at or spoke to you in a certain way. I was growing more nervous every day.

With the very poor outcomes we were seeing for barrel-bomb victims, we had to find something to latch on to that was positive. I managed to continue with some teaching, especially vascular work with Abu Hozaifa, and more training with Abu Waseem, the only plastic surgeon in Aleppo. Many of our cases required fairly simple reconstructive surgery but it was life-changing for those we operated on, and one little boy offered a glimmer of hope. He was brought in following a barrel-bomb injury to his left leg. He was on his own, without any family. He was silent on the operating table. Many children are like this—often because they have lost a lot of blood, but in some cases they are simply mute from the psychological trauma.

I went to see him and it was obvious that he had a significant leg injury. The fragment had taken all the skin from the lower leg and foot, and at the same time had destroyed all three blood vessels supplying that area. It would have been very easy to simply go for an amputation, but that would have left him with a pretty miserable life ahead. So Ammar, Abu Hozaifa, Abu Waseem, and I decided to do our best to salvage his leg.

It was a major challenge. A four-year-old's blood vessels are very small, and the chances of success even in a state-of-the-art operating facility would probably be equally tiny. I got my favorite anesthesiologist, Mohammed Wehybi, to put him to sleep. He was the nineteen-year-old anesthesiology technician who had been working in Aleppo the year before. He was absolutely amazing. He could put intravenous lines in people with collapsed veins and seemed able to put anybody to sleep safely. He put the little boy under and I proceeded to take the long saphenous vein, the superficial vein, from the boy's right leg to use as a bypass graft. I dissected out the artery below the knee and carefully joined the vein to this artery, using the finest sutures we could find. The vein graft was then plumbed onto a tiny artery near the foot. When the clamps came off, I was pleased to see the foot begin to pink up. This part of the operation had been a success and we put some very light dressings onto the leg and took the boy back to the ward. I worried, though, that the overall procedure would fail, because the trauma to the leg was so serious.

The following day we brought him back to the operating room and again put him to sleep. I was delighted that the bypass graft seemed to be functioning beautifully—despite having had a lot of skin removed, his foot was now warm, as were his toes. Next we had to cover as much of the skin of the lower leg and foot as we could. The only option here was to perform a cross-leg flap. This procedure involves taking skin and fascia, which lines the muscles of the lower leg, and making it into a big sheet of skin that can then be stitched onto the injured leg.

I taught Abu Waseem how to do this and we raised the flap and stitched it over the vein graft on the other leg. It was important that the two legs were kept together to allow the blood vessels from the injured leg to grow into the cross-leg flap and provide its circulation. To do this, we used orthopedic external fixators to join the boy's little legs together. We took him back to the ward and constructed a sort of hoist that allowed him to be fed and have his bottom wiped. He would be stuck in this position for about three weeks. So far, so good.

By this point, Castello Road was under attack, and Ammar told me that he'd heard it was now closed to all vehicles going in and out of Aleppo. If the road really had been closed by the regime, we were stuck. It left me feeling frightened and exposed. I began to feel I didn't know who or what was around me. All I knew for certain was that the only people I could trust were Ammar and a few other close Syrian colleagues.

A few hours after hearing this news, I happened to be in M2, having operated upon a sick child there. I was downstairs waiting for Ammar, who had left my side for a few minutes, one of the very few occasions that he did so. While I was sitting there on my own, a surgeon whom I had met a couple of times before but didn't really know sidled up to me and said he thought my surgical skills would be better used with ISIS in Raqqa. Did I want to go and work with them there?

"Er, no thanks, I'm all right here."

"If you want to go, I can arrange it all," he persisted, waggling his cell phone.

I should have stayed silent, or smiled and said I'd think about it, but all my anxiety and frustration boiled over and I began to tell him how disgusted I was at the very idea. Just as the argument was really getting going, Ammar returned.

"Be careful, David," he whispered in my ear. "Be very careful."

I knew the risks, of course, but I couldn't help expressing my revulsion, and was by now so strung out I felt I had nothing to lose. As the mission neared its end the pain in my chest became more and more intense, and every 3:00 a.m. knock on the door of our bedroom produced a massive adrenaline rush, as I wondered whether the knock was someone calling me to see a patient or coming to take me away. When the final knock came, it was Abu Mohammadain, who had come to tell Ammar and me that there was a very small window of opportunity to get us out. We'd had no fixed day of departure, just a general feeling that if Castello Road was clear it was time to go.

We left on Friday morning at 5:30, just as the sun was coming up. Abu Waseem said he would accompany us. We had word from Bab al-Hawa that they had many patients in need of reconstructive surgery, and Abu Waseem was going to operate on them. Abu Hozaifa said he wanted to come, too. I wanted to bring the little boy with us, so that we could attend to his wounds. There were two cars, with me and Ammar in the back of one, while the man who had brought us in with his heavy body armor and helmet and weapons sat next to Abu Mohammadain, who was driving. Abu Hozaifa, Abu Waseem, and the little boy were in the second car. It might seem odd that we wanted him to endure such a dangerous journey, but he needed his wounds tending twice a day and without Abu Waseem to do that, the chances of the procedure succeeding were slim. We had got so far with him, it was only right to give him the very best chance we could.

We approached the outskirts of the city. Ahead of us was an obstacle course of bullet-ridden and overturned cars, some of which had been bravely pushed to one side so that the road was still passable. We had to traverse about two miles of the most dangerous road in the world: the regime's guns were probably less than a hundred meters to the right, while to the left were the rebels.

Abu Mohammadain stopped the car where it was still safe. He looked around at us and reached out and shook our hands. I knew, as did Ammar, that what he was saying was goodbye. Ammar said, "David, you OK to go?" I pursed my lips and nodded. The situation was so desperate that the risk was worth it. The drivers in both cars nodded at each other, and then Abu Mohammadain floored it, so we were going at top speed by the time we reached the obstacles. How we got through those gaps I will never know—the car seemed to be skidding and sliding all over the place at breakneck speed. But we did it, we got through, and not a shot was fired.

The rest of the drive north was a walk in the park; even the threat of regime jets targeting us seemed pretty minor. We arrived at Bab al-Hawa and spent the next three days operating nonstop, trying to get through the backlog of patients needing reconstructive work. All four of us—Ammar, Abu Hozaifa, Abu Waseem, and myself—acted as a kind of surgical conveyor-belt until we had achieved our goal. We checked in regularly on our little boy, who seemed to be doing well. Amazingly the cross-leg flap was still working, the arterial bypass graft was doing its job, and he was not septic.

All four of us stayed in a little room in a safe house next to the hospital. On our last day the ICU specialist Ammar Zacharia turned up—somehow he'd known we were there, and he said he was going to arrange a fruit festival as a gift to us. I'd never heard of a fruit festival, but later that afternoon he arrived bearing fresh bananas, apples, oranges, and all sorts of fruit arrayed on a huge platter.

As we dug in, it was as though an enormous weight had lifted from our shoulders. But as ever with this mission, there was a sting in the tail. Suddenly, we heard the sound of heavy gunfire outside the house. I peered through a crack in the window and could see about twenty armed men coming toward us, some walking and firing their weapons, others with heavy-caliber machine guns on the back of pickup trucks. It seemed I was fated not to leave Syria. If Ammar Zacharia had found out we were there, so could others. Had ISIS finally caught up with me? I looked at Ammar and for the first time he looked really scared, his face white with fear.

I began to panic. I was cold and clammy and began shaking uncontrollably. The fighting outside intensified. We hit the deck, hiding under our beds. I wondered if I should try to get out and disappear, and whispered as much to Ammar. To my mind this would serve two purposes—first, the others wouldn't be tarnished by association with me; and second, it might give me a better chance of survival than being caught in this room by ISIS. But the only way out was the front door, and it would be impossible to leave without being seen. So I just closed my eyes and lay there, in despair—for myself, and for this poor country that had been overwhelmed by darkness.

The shooting lasted around an hour, with the Free Syrian Army firing from positions all around us. At some point Munzer, the hospital administrator, managed to get into our room and told me, quite nonchalantly, that I was not to worry—the fighting was just between two rival FSA factions.

It turned out later he had hidden the reality of the situation to protect me. The fighters *were* ISIS, and it was their last chance to take me hostage—Munzer confessed the truth six months later, at a medical conference in Turkey. I thanked him for his white lie—if I had known this at the time, the stress would undoubtedly have killed me. A few hours later, after the fighting had stopped, Ammar and I crossed into Turkey. We had said our goodbyes to Abu Hozaifa and Abu Waseem—they were staying with the little boy for a few more days, before going back to Aleppo if the road was still open.

No sooner had we crossed the border than my phone pinged. I had been sent a photo via WhatsApp of Mohammed Wehybi, the best anesthesiologist in Aleppo, lying in a shroud, killed by a barrel bomb while traveling from one hospital to another. But I was too numb to grieve. Death had become all too routine.

Once we had reached the Syria Relief office in Reyhanlı, I first spoke to Ghanem Tayara, the head of UOSSM, the Union of Medical Care and Relief Organizations. It was obvious that he was hugely relieved that we had got out unharmed. I could tell from his voice that he had been on tenterhooks.

My second call was to Elly. We had barely spoken for six weeks. It was strange, and wonderful, to be talking to her again, and I was so happy that she still seemed to care for me. But I was no longer sure who I was. The mission had taken me apart. I was not sure if Elly would have the appetite, or the ability, to put me back together.

- 12 -
PHYSICIAN, HEAL THYSELF

Ammar and I stayed together for the day in Reyhanlı and went for a quiet meal, our moods very different from the elation of the year before. He asked me what I was going to do after I got back to the UK. Bizarrely, the only thing I could think of, apart from seeing Elly, was swimming. I wanted to walk across a beach and wade deeper and deeper into the sea, until the waves broke over my head. A desire to be cleansed, perhaps to wash away the dreadful things I'd witnessed, and begin again, like some kind of baptism.

The bit of coastline I knew best was at St. Andrews in Scotland, where I'd gone to university. I had loved my time there, and felt a strong desire to reconnect with a place that had only good memories. I also wanted to show Elly something of who I was, where I'd come from. I came out of arrivals at Heathrow and there she was, standing calm and still amid the hurly-burly of the airport, having waited hours for me to come. The next morning we boarded a plane to Edinburgh and then hired a car to go on to St. Andrews, where I had booked a room at a very grand hotel. My bank account was decidedly in the red, but I didn't care.

It was a wonderful few days and I was relieved that the enforced separation and lack of contact while I'd been in Syria seemed to have made no difference in how we felt about each other. Elly instinctively seemed to know how to take my mind off the death and destruction of Aleppo. On our last night I sprang the idea of a swim on her. It was mid-October, and dark, with a gale-force wind blowing along the West Sands as we walked down to the shore. I knew it was crazy but it was something I needed to do. I wanted to blow away the memories of barrel bombs and dust and silent children. Turning to face her, I told Elly that she didn't need to come in with me. "Wherever you go, I will go too," she replied. We took off our clothes and ran into the sea. It was pitch-black, with only the occasional glimmer of light on the waves, and freezing cold. We waded forward blindly until we felt the water lapping at our thighs and then plunged in. I felt alive again.

It was then that I decided that Elly was the woman I wanted to spend the rest of my life with.

We left Scotland and went back to normality. Except things weren't normal. Often, when I'd returned from difficult missions before, I had been aware that my behavior was different for a while as I decompressed and readjusted to London life and work. I was taught by my parents to be courteous and respectful to everybody, and to always look for the best in people. But following a particularly difficult mission, there is no doubt my personality sometimes changed, and I became more irritable and aggressive, as was sometimes pointed out to me by colleagues.

Very rarely, this post-mission stress would manifest in some kind of outburst. I remember sitting in my office the day after I got back from that horrendous mission to the Chad-Darfur border, where we lost so many patients and babies during very difficult Cesarean sections, and had no spare blood and few supplies. I was exhausted from the physical work, and brutalized by the psychological trauma of seeing so much suffering. As ever, it was the children that had really got to me.

It was probably not the most sensible time to be doing a private outpatients' session—the problems I was dealing with in my room off Sloane Square all seemed pointless and trivial. I nodded my way through, on autopilot, but by mid-afternoon I could feel myself getting ever more tense and angry.

The penultimate patient of the day was asking me where I had been in the world. I told her that I had just come back from Darfur, and that it had been particularly difficult. She was worried about her spider veins, which she thought looked unsightly, and I was injecting her with a drug that causes these superficial veins to shrivel up. You must have taken an awful lot of bottles of this drug with you to Africa, she said, to treat all those poor people who had spider veins. It wasn't her fault, of course, that she didn't understand what I had been doing there, but it was the catalyst for what happened next.

My final patient came in. She was very, very unhappy that she had had to wait for six weeks to see me, and very, very disappointed that I did not seem to care that she had been made to wait. She began talking about her problem, which again seemed to me utterly trivial. As she was talking all I could hear was a roaring in my ears; I could see her jaw flapping up and down as she yammered on but I could not hear a word she was saying, just the roaring and roaring as the tension in my body rose until I couldn't take it any longer. I suddenly stood up and screamed as loudly as I could.

She looked at me in astonishment. "What on earth is the matter?"

"Aaaaggghh!" I screamed again, clutching at my right thigh and staggering around the room pretending to be in complete agony. I had to get rid of her before I told her to fuck off out of my consulting room.

"It's my sciatica," I gasped as I fell onto the sofa, "terrible sciatica."

"Oh my goodness; do you think I should go?"

"Yes—aaaahhh, ohhh, the pain—yes, I'm afraid so."

I opened the door, saying I was in too much pain to continue, and that she could make another appointment next month as I probably needed to be admitted to hospital.

With that, she left, and I sat on my consulting room chair for the next three hours just staring at the ceiling.

Thankfully, episodes like this were very rare, and most of the time I was able to rationalize my situation, certain that it would all be fine in the end. And it always was. But it was a long way from fine now. Over the last ten months a lot had happened. I had had a painful mission to Africa; I'd been to Gaza, where I had had to confront not only my own mortality but also the fact that my life seemed devoid of anyone who would notice if I died. And I'd been back to Syria, where innocent civilians and children were subjected to horrendous violence, while the world largely ignored it.

I was not in a good place. My diminishing ability to cope was rather spectacularly exposed quite soon after my return, when I was invited to a private lunch with the Queen at Buckingham Palace. I am not sure how this came about; I knew the broadcast of my Eddie Mair interview had touched a lot of people, so perhaps someone in the royal household had also tuned in. In any event, one day not long after I got back I put on my one and only suit and waved goodbye to Elly as I passed through the gates of the Palace.

The contrast between those gilded walls and the ravaged streets of Aleppo began doing weird things to my head. I walked along the red carpet into one of the reception rooms and stood awkwardly with the other guests. I felt a fraud, guilty—I should not be here enjoying this splendor and warm hospitality while my friends in Aleppo are suffering. I looked at the seating plan and found that I was sitting on the Queen's left, which I knew was an honor. But I was perilously close to a panic attack.

I stood dumbly with the other guests making small talk with Prince Philip. God knows what he must have thought. Finally we were taken through to the dining room and one of the courtiers showed me to my seat next to the Queen. Etiquette dictates that the Queen will speak to the person on her right for half the lunch and will then turn to the person on her left for the second half. I realize now that I should have been speaking first to the person on my left, but I cannot recall doing so and whoever it was must have thought me extremely rude. I could feel myself staring into space.

The dessert arrived and the Queen turned to me. At first I couldn't hear what she was saying, as my hearing had been damaged by a bomb blast near the hospital in Aleppo. I tried to speak, but nothing would come out of my mouth. It wasn't that I didn't want to speak to her; I couldn't. I simply did not know what to say.

She asked me where had I come from. I suppose she was expecting me to say, "From Hammersmith," or something like that, but I told her I had recently returned from Aleppo.

"Oh," she said. "And what was that like?"

What was it like? What could I say? My mind filled instantly with images of toxic dust, of crushed school desks, of bloodied and limbless children. And of Alan Henning and those other Westerners whose lives had ended in the most appalling fashion.

I don't know why it happened then, or why it should have been the Queen who breached the dam. Perhaps it was because she is the mother of the nation, and I had lost my own mother. My bottom lip started to go and all I wanted to do was to burst into tears, but I held myself together as best I could. I hoped she wouldn't ask me another question about Aleppo. I knew if she did, I would completely lose control.

She looked at me quizzically and touched my hand. She then had a quiet word with one of the courtiers, who pointed to a silver box in front of her. I watched as she opened the box, which was full of biscuits. "These are for the dogs," she said, breaking one of the biscuits in two and giving me half. We fed the biscuits to the corgis under the table, and for the rest of the lunch she took the lead and chatted about her dogs, how many she had, what their names were, how old they were. All the while we were stroking and petting them, and my anxiety and distress drained away.

"There," the Queen said. "That's so much better than talking, isn't it?"

Queen Elizabeth's instinctive insight into my emotional fragility was remarkable, as was the compassion she showed toward somebody she had never met. But although an embarrassing scene had been narrowly averted, it did not change the fact that I was not well.

I found myself being aggravated by the smallest things, arguing about nothing. I felt detached from the world around me, like someone who had no understanding of reality. My behavior became increasingly irrational. I flew into rages and suffered from a general and persistent sense of desperation.

Elly was very supportive of what I was going through but could see that I wasn't my normal self, and, of course, it got to her. I remember one day she had bought herself a lovely dress. We were out together that evening and she became so distraught at how I was behaving she just sat down on the dirty pavement in her new outfit, put her head in her hands, and wept. I remember thinking, *What have I done?* but I couldn't change the emotional rollercoaster I was on, and just stood there looking at her like some lumpen ogre.

Over Christmas we went skiing in Chamonix. How apt that the room we were allocated was number 101—in George Orwell's novel *Nineteen Eighty-Four*, Room 101 is a torture chamber in the Ministry of Love in which the all-powerful Party subjects prisoners to their worst nightmares. I don't know whether it was the altitude or my state of mind, but in that room I slipped into a trough of psychosis and paranoia.

Poor Elly—she had to put up with a lot. I would lie in front of the door in a fetal position, unable to move, observing myself as if from a distance and watching Elly become more and more distraught. I was confrontational and critical of every aspect of her character. I thought she had become my jailer, my executioner, and that I needed to stop her from leaving the room. This went on for days, and I almost lost her.

Somehow, despite the depths of my psychosis, I knew that I had to talk to someone, and once we were back in London, I went to see a psychiatrist I knew. He was very helpful, not only listening as I tearfully unburdened myself for hours, but also offering some tough love. "Get a grip," he said. "Stop behaving like an arse, and be kind to her." Of course, this was pretty much Elly's own diagnosis, but for some reason I needed to hear it from someone else.

Through much of my life I had felt alone. It was completely irrational that the person who showed me so much love, showed me the way to live a different kind of life, should be the person I was most angry with. I had never felt such love for anyone before, yet I seemed to want to push her away.

It's tempting to think of my breakdown as being caused by the cumulative effect of the stresses I had experienced over the years—the brushes with death, the danger, the constant emotional assault of seeing innocent people and children suffer. But I'd always been able to move on in the past. What was different now? Was it that 2014 had been particularly difficult, culminating in that brutal mission to barrel-bombed Aleppo? Perhaps. But I think the main difference was Elly. Before, I had had nothing to come back to; now, I did—and, in some ways, it was terrifying. There was so much more at stake now.

With help, I began to deal with my problems. I had a course of cognitive behavioral therapy and antipsychotic drugs were suggested, although in the end they proved unnecessary. With Elly's remarkable patience and forbearance, I was rescued from myself.

As I got better, and my demons retreated to the shadows, the world continued to turn and the occasional call continued to come in. Given that I had been banned from MSF since Atmeh in 2012, I was surprised to hear from them one day in late April 2015. They wanted me to go to Arughat Bazar in Nepal, which was near the epicenter of an earthquake that had killed some

9,000 people and injured over 20,000 more. They needed an answer within hours. If it was yes, I would be on a plane later that day.

But things were different now. Elly and I were married. And not only that, just ten days before our wedding I was in the shower when Elly came into the bathroom and told me to get out immediately. She handed me a pregnancy-test stick, which was clearly positive.

Although Nepal was not a war zone, it was a challenging environment and one not easy to get to or back from. However, I still had the same visceral reaction to a request for help. I tried to suppress the urge to go, and in fact refused their request. But then they called again: there had been a second quake, a big aftershock, and they really needed help. I had to go. I made a very difficult telephone call to Elly, who was at first shocked and upset but by the time we were saying our goodbyes she was as steadfast and supportive as she always is.

After arriving in Kathmandu I found myself in a car that took seven hours negotiating landslides and crevasses to get to one of MSF's inflatable hospitals. Many of the injuries had been dealt with before I got there, and I found myself being not a trauma surgeon at all, but an obstetrician. As I got out of the car, exhausted from the long journey, a midwife ran up, saying, "Thank God you're here, there's an obstructed breech and we need you right now, there's a foot hanging out of the vagina!" To my delight and relief I saw that Rachel Craven was the anesthesiologist; within a few moments she had given the patient a spinal block and I performed a lower segment Cesarean section, delivering the baby bottom first.

On my return, Elly and I had a long talk. She had realized that my urge to volunteer in such situations was almost beyond my control; it would be part of our life together. But with a baby on the way, we agreed my new responsibilities as a husband and father might affect *where* I went.

While I was away Elly had also made progress on a project that I had wanted to develop for years, but had neither the time nor the knowledge to implement. I had known for some time that the Surgical Training for Austere Environments course at the Royal College of Surgeons would be so much more effective if we could somehow sponsor surgeons from all over the world to attend. But we'd need money, which meant raising funds. We needed to set up a charity. Through Elly's diligence and hard work, the David Nott Foundation was awarded charitable status in July 2015.

And that month brought another birth—the arrival of our first child, Molly, who was born nine months to the day after my return from Syria. People often describe becoming a parent as the best day of their life, and with good reason; the world around you is configured anew. You are no longer the endpoint of a genetic chain, but merely a link along it. Elly and I were surrounded by friends and colleagues with whom I had worked for twenty years at the Chelsea and Westminster Hospital, including Mark Johnson, who was the obstetrician, and Mark Cox, the anesthesiologist—by this time I think he'd forgiven me for almost killing him in the helicopter. It was a magical experience, and has remained so ever since, as was the birth of Molly's sister, Elizabeth Rose, who joined our little family some twenty months later.

Now that the foundation is up and running, surgeons from all over the world can apply for scholarships that pay the course fees and all travel and accommodation costs. They return home full of new techniques and as much information as possible to provide improved care for their patients. We have also developed a satellite course called the Hostile Environment Surgical Training course (HEST), which can be taken to the front line for surgeons in the field who are unable to leave their post. Over the past two years we have used it to train Syrian surgeons on the Turkey-Syria border, and in Yemen, the West Bank, Gaza, Libya, Iraq, and Cameroon. So far, we have trained more than seven hundred local surgeons.

This expertise is needed more than ever. Russia entered the Syrian conflict at the end of September 2015, at the request of the beleaguered Assad regime. The original justification was to strike at ISIS in Syria, but there was no doubt that they were there to prop up the regime. Assad's forces had been struggling and had already been bolstered by militias from Iran and Hezbollah. It suited Russia to be involved. By standing up to the West, President Putin could challenge the decades-long US monopoly of influence in the Middle East.

In March 2016 I took three weeks off work to go back to the border region, to a small hospital in Reyhanlı where patients were allowed to cross from Syria for treatment. Many of these cases moved me to tears, even while I was examining them in the emergency room. Because of Molly, I felt even more emotionally connected to the children I saw. One little girl had been involved in an airstrike a few months before, and she had such severe burns that she had lost both her hands and her face was very badly damaged. Her parents brought her into the outpatients' clinic in a stroller with an umbrella over it so that nobody could see her. Her parents showed me a picture of her before the attack. She looked just like Molly. It was heartbreaking.

On July 19, 2016, Castello Road was finally closed and east Aleppo was entirely surrounded by government forces. Meanwhile Abu Waseem was sending me WhatsApp videos and pictures of cases he wanted me to help him with. I advised where I could, but it was a litany of suffering, and he was clearly affected by the thanklessness of the task. One day he sent me two photos of a young child with horrific injuries. "Look at this girl," he wrote. "This is one of the victims of a Russian bombing today. She lost her whole arm and her face."

"Terrible," I replied. "Is she going to survive?"

"Unfortunately, yes."

The latest threat was from chemical weapons—he told me he'd recently had around twenty patients admitted following a chlorine attack. His emergency room was full, and he didn't have enough masks or oxygen cylinders to treat them all. Two patients subsequently died from the chlorine, which reacts with water and turns into hydrochloric acid, dissolving the lungs of anyone unfortunate enough to inhale it.

A week later I heard from Abu Mohammadain, who was still working in M10. He sent me a picture of a little boy he had been treating. A video showing the bloodied face of this shocked and petrified child had gone viral on social media and was on all the news channels. The little boy obviously did not understand what was going on around him. He had sustained a severe gash to his scalp and blood was pouring down his face. He sat on his own in the ambulance staring vacantly into space. No one knew where his parents were.

The next day Abu Waseem messaged me with news that the little boy's brother had been admitted to M1. He had sustained a severe liver injury and had died on the operating table. Waseem was obviously devastated. How had things got so bad? Where was it going to end? I was becoming more and more anguished and outraged.

When President Obama had talked in 2013 about "crossing the red line" after four hundred children were killed by a chemical weapons attack in Ghouta, outside Damascus, he was awaiting the outcome of a vote on military action in the British Parliament. The vote was close, but in the end 285 Members of Parliament (MPs) against 272 decided not to proceed with strikes against the Syrian regime. Unfortunately the debate seemed to be more about politicking between the prime minister, David Cameron, and the leader of the opposition, Ed Miliband, rather than what was the right thing to do. It was, in some ways, a reaction to Tony Blair's support for the US invasion of Iraq a decade earlier. The aftermath of that war has left a toxic legacy: the British people just didn't want to become embroiled in someone else's war in a faraway place of which they knew very little. But I have no doubt that if the West had shown strong leadership at that point, the Syrian military hierarchy would have collapsed.

Following the 2013 Ghouta attack, Assad's regime acknowledged possession of chemical weapons and agreed to be put under international supervision endorsed by UN Security Council Resolution 2118. (The deadline for the destruction of their chemical weapons stockpile was the first half of 2014, and they claimed then to have complied. However, attacks at Khan Shaykhun in April 2017 and Douma in April 2018 revealed that they had been either lying or restocking.) Meanwhile, Abu Waseem continued to text me to let me know that there were clouds of chlorine gas being dropped in barrel bombs around his hospital, and the number of attacks was increasing by the day.

At the end of August 2016 he contacted me to ask if I'd be able to help them with a patient who had a severe facial injury following a barrel-bomb attack. He was a thirty-five-year-old father of three, several of whose friends had been killed in the same attack. His mouth and the lower part of his jaw were hanging free and there was a significant risk of him developing an infection. They had done all they could, but wanted to know whether

I could help them reconstruct the man's jaw. Amazingly, they had had a CT scanner built in M10, and sent me pictures of his face via WhatsApp.

I showed the pictures to several colleagues who were experts in facio-maxillary work. The patient had been left with only the two struts of his jawbone on either side, attached to the temporomandibular joints—the joints between the upper jaw and head.

Ask ten different surgeons their opinion and you get ten different answers. It was a difficult call, to be fair—some surgeons said that reconstruction was impossible; others suggested the only way would be to use a free flap from the leg, including one of the leg bones, and use a microscope to join up the very small arteries and veins. I had the idea of using a metal plate, fashioning it into a semicircle so it could be joined to the two remaining bones by screws, thus completing the outline of the jaw. The metal plate would then be covered by a muscle to reconstruct the floor of the mouth, and the front of the mouth would be covered by skin that would be attached to the muscle, the so-called myocutaneous flap. It would be a major undertaking at the best of times. The concept of doing it remotely, with me directing things from London, was unprecedented.

We decided to give it a try, using a muscle flap and skin from the pectoralis major muscle, which is supplied by an artery below the collarbone, and then rotate that with an appropriate patch of skin to cover the new lower jaw. Abu Waseem and his colleagues were very excited. They had a week to scour through the remaining hospitals and rubble for the correct sterile plate and screws. In the meantime I sent over as much information as I could regarding the technique.

The day before the operation we had one last Skype conversation and it was confirmed that they had two units of blood available for the procedure. As it happened, I had been asked about the situation in Aleppo by BBC Two's *Newsnight* program and told them I was about to oversee a challenging operation there via Skype. They agreed to record the procedure, and share with the world the remarkable courage of Aleppo's besieged doctors.

So there I was in London, looking at a large television screen. The patient was asleep on the operating table at M10 in Aleppo. We set up the Skype call and someone in the operating room put an iPhone on a selfie stick that was held over the table, so I could see everything that was going on during the operation. Because the surgeons had never done this procedure before, I began directing proceedings. First, they screwed the metal plate into what remained of the two struts of the jawbone, which took about two hours. Then we came to the most difficult part of the procedure. The pectoralis major muscle is the broad muscle that lies on the anterior chest wall below the nipple. Because they had never mobilized this muscle and didn't know exactly where to make the incisions, I first of all asked them to raise a deltopectoral flap, by lifting a large piece of skin below the collarbone from the chest to expose the whole of the pectoralis major muscle. This took about another hour. Meanwhile, we took lots of measurements to confirm that the muscle and skin would actually rotate underneath the metal plate into the bottom of the mouth and jaw.

We proceeded with the operation and I directed them exactly where to make the incisions. Over the next six hours they mobilized the correct amount of muscle with the correct amount of skin and by the end of the day had successfully completed the operation. It was the most extraordinary achievement.

A few days later, the report went out on *Newsnight* and it can still be seen on YouTube. Apart from helping the patient, it elevated the doctors' mood—they took hope from the knowledge that people all over the world had seen what was happening. Abu Waseem and his colleagues continued to let me know how the patient progressed. When the doctors at M10 removed the patient's tracheotomy tube, he began to cry, saying, "God bless you all." I was thrilled to have been able to help both my colleagues and the patient. It was a ray of hope in the darkness of war.

In September, however, the situation deteriorated dramatically. In the last weekend of that month I had around a hundred WhatsApp messages from my Syrian colleagues. They had received 168 casualties in just a few hours, following barrel bombs and constant airstrikes throughout the day. Of those, around half were children, and there were many other deaths unaccounted for. It appeared that people had been queueing for food at the market when a squadron of fighters came in firing rockets. As well as rockets, government forces and the Russians were also dropping cluster bombs, and bigger devices called bunker-busting bombs, which drilled a hole on impact with the ground and then exploded several feet below the surface, thus killing people who were hiding in the basements of their houses. The hospitals were also receiving casualties who had what appeared to be ball-bearings deeply implanted in their bodies. It was horrendous. I was desperately anxious not only for my colleagues but for all the civilians and innocent children who were being slowly annihilated.

I wanted to do something as quickly as I could to encourage politicians to try to stop this disaster from getting any worse. Elly suggested that I go and see Andrew Mitchell, who was one of the most vocal MPs on humanitarian matters and who had done good work when he was Her Majesty's Principal Secretary of State for International Development. Surprisingly, he agreed to meet me. We discussed the situation that was unfolding and how the civilians left in east Aleppo were being pounded every day by Syrian and Russian jets. I showed him photographs of dead and dying children that I had been sent and suggested that the British government really needed to step in to try and stop the carnage.

I embarked upon a media offensive as well, appearing on radio and television whenever I could to talk about what was happening, and the risk the doctors were facing—a risk which was brought home horribly in early October, just a few weeks after the successful Skype operation. I was sent a WhatsApp video of a bunker-busting bomb dropping directly onto the operating room in M10. The target was so precise that the coordinates of the OR must have been known. I could only think, to my horror, that somebody must have hacked the Skype call and somehow deduced M10's location. In the minutes after the bunker bomb fell, a further three barrel bombs and two cluster bombs were dropped on M10. At the time, the hospital's intensive care unit was full, the wards were full, and the recovery unit was full. The hospital was destroyed; many patients died and the survivors were moved to surrounding hospitals, which also came under attack. But, amazingly, all my surgical colleagues were still alive.

On October 5, a UN convoy that had taken a good deal of diplomacy to organize was about to deliver medical aid and food into east Aleppo when it came under attack from the air and was wiped out. Both the Russian and

Syrian air forces denied responsibility. Five days later Matthew Rycroft, the UK's ambassador to the UN, delivered a damning speech to the Security Council condemning unprecedented Russian-backed shelling in the war in Syria, saying that the country's pretensions to peace in the country were a sham. The Russian representative had vetoed a draft resolution to revive the ceasefire and end airstrikes, except those against ISIS and al-Qaeda-affiliated rebels in Syria. It was the fifth time that Russia had used its position as a permanent member of the Security Council to block UN action over Syria.

As all this was going on, Andrew Mitchell had applied to the Speaker of the House of Commons for an emergency debate under Standing Order 24. The debate went ahead on October 11 and Elly and I sat in the gallery to watch. Many good people spoke, but the chamber was not full and at the end we walked away feeling very disappointed. However, it did start the ball rolling in the sense that at least Parliament was now talking about the atrocities in Aleppo. Until then, I'd had the feeling that MPs just didn't want to know.

Over the next few days another four hundred civilians died and thousands of others were injured. Several more hospitals were put out of action. The Aleppo City Medical Council was reaching a breaking point because of the volume of casualties and their dwindling resources. They finally made a formal request to the UN for the injured to be evacuated and humanitarian aid to be delivered. But because of the previous attacks on convoys, their requests fell on deaf ears.

In late October I returned to Syria, with Mounir, to Bab al-Hawa Hospital, to operate on some of the wounded who had been caught up in the heavy shelling around Aleppo. The Syrian regime claimed to have made safe corridors available to people who wanted to leave east Aleppo, but no one took them up on the offer because they didn't trust the assurances of safe passage.

For the next two weeks there was a reduction in the number of airstrikes, and although food and medical supplies were dwindling, the message out of Aleppo seemed more optimistic. I wondered whether international pressure was finally making a difference. But then the stakes were raised again. In mid-November regime leaflets rained down from the sky telling people that they had twenty-four hours to leave via the supposedly safe corridors, or they would suffer the effects of a huge offensive on east Aleppo. The following day there were nearly two hundred airstrikes and as many artillery shells, killing hundreds of civilians. The children's hospital was destroyed. But still people stayed—they didn't want to leave their homes, and they worried that as soon as they surrendered themselves to the care of Assad's regime, they would be arrested, or worse.

On my return, I found myself writing in every newspaper and appearing on every television and radio channel that would have me. We had to get these people out, I argued, and via routes that they could trust, not those organized or supervised by the Syrian government. But how? It seemed an impossible task—the brutal dance of Syria and Russia in Aleppo held the city in a vise. Where could we even begin?

- 13 -
ESCAPE FROM ALEPPO

Over the next few weeks I found myself sucked into a bizarre shadow-world of international diplomacy and back-channel negotiations. The siege of Aleppo became harder and harder to endure—the assault from the regime intensified, and the small enclave still held by rebel forces, where my friends worked, shrank almost by the day. Casualty numbers escalated, supplies dwindled, and the perils increased.

I wanted to help the people of Aleppo more broadly, but I am not a miracle worker and it was impossible to think in terms of tens of thousands. It was hard enough thinking about my thirty or so medical colleagues, the people I knew personally and had worked with. I found it easier to focus my thoughts on just one man: my friend Abu Waseem. I was determined to get Abu Waseem safely out of east Aleppo. If others managed to make it out with him, so much the better.

I have always had a tendency to focus on specific tasks and pursue them relentlessly, sometimes flying in the face of all logic or common sense. Dogged determination, I suppose. Getting Landina's passport in Haiti was one example. Another is something that happened when I was a young consultant, and which perhaps set the pattern for the years that followed.

I was working at Charing Cross Hospital and I was called to the emergency room to see a young woman who had fallen in the gap between the platform and a train at Hammersmith station. She had been trying to pull herself up onto the platform when the train started to move. Her pelvis was trapped and as the train pulled away, it rotated her pelvis and legs almost 180° while her body remained upright.

I walked into the emergency room wearing the smart new suit my mother had bought me to go with my new job as a consultant, and was faced with a young woman bleeding to death. Her name was Yvette, and she had been anesthetized at the scene and was on a ventilator. She needed immediate surgery. Her blood pressure was dangerously low, around 40 systolic. The team in the ER was quickly setting up drips, but if I had waited for them to finish she would surely have died. I took my jacket off, rolled up my shirtsleeves, and asked for a pair of sterile gloves and a knife. I needed to stop the bleeding, and stop it immediately. I knew I had to clamp her aorta, and took the quickest route, somewhat to the surprise of everyone present. Admittedly, it must have seemed quite a drastic move. I made a midline incision from the breastbone to the pubis without using any antiseptic and swiftly put a cross clamp on the aorta. I could see that her pelvis was a complete mess—but that was something to fix later, once the blood pressure had come back up.

My new pants and shoes were covered in blood and I ended up losing my jacket in all the confusion. I quickly put on scrubs in the surgeons' changing room and went into surgery. She had injuries to her ureters, bladder, vagina, and uterus, and all her major arteries and veins had been damaged. During the rotation of her pelvis, a spicule of bone from the pelvic skeleton had sliced through her pelvic organs and major blood vessels.

I needed help. I called a consultant urologist whom I respected greatly, Jonathan Ramsay, and also asked the on-call orthopedic surgeon to stabilize her pelvis. By this time, with as many clamps on as many bleeding arteries and veins as I could find, I had stemmed most of the bleeding. The orthopedic surgeon proceeded to fixate the pelvis externally, while Jonathan and I debated what we should do. There were huge rents—the medical term for tear—extending into the uterus and bladder, and blood was pouring from these organs. The ureters, which take urine from the kidney to the bladder, were also damaged and in urgent need of Jonathan's technical expertise. We had an agonizing discussion about whether she should have a hysterectomy. Should we take the uterus out and be done with it, or should we try to preserve it? If we kept the uterus and she died, it would be dreadful, but if she lived, she might be able to have children. Both options carried great risks.

Jonathan sutured her organs back together again while I sutured her blood vessels and reestablished arterial flow to her pelvis and legs. We stitched and stitched and stitched for several hours until all the bleeding had ceased.

But she was still desperately ill. Apart from all her other problems, she had a degloving injury to her pelvis—that is, when the skin is physically removed from the underlying tissue. She went to the intensive care unit at around seven in the evening but, given the extent of her injuries, we felt she had only a 10 percent chance of surviving the night.

It was then that I found myself on a path from which I could not deviate. I decided that she would not die on my watch. Every hour, on the hour, throughout the night, I packed her various bleeding points with gauze, changing them when they were sodden with blood. At nine the following morning I was exhausted, but she was still alive.

Over the next three months Yvette went back and forth to the operating room for more plastic-surgical and urological procedures while still in the intensive care unit, under the watchful eye of Mark Palazzo, the director of the ICU. She was eventually discharged home after several months on the ward, to her amazingly supportive family and boyfriend, soon to be her fiancé. Two years later, I sat in church with Jonathan, moved to tears, as we watched Yvette walk up the aisle on her father's arm. It was a moment to cherish—as it was when we heard she was expecting her first child.

That stubborn refusal to countenance that Yvette might die had stayed with me. And I was similarly determined now in the case of Abu Waseem. He and his colleagues were seriously worried about how they'd be treated by the Syrian government if they availed themselves of their offers of safe passage out of eastern Aleppo. They knew all too well what happened to those who were thought to have aided the rebels. There had to be another way out. But it would probably need United Nations help, and almost certainly a ceasefire, which would have to be agreed with Assad's regime. But why would they agree? And who would persuade them? They might listen to pressure from the Russians, but whether the Russians could be persuaded to make the case was by no means certain. And UN support for such a plan was not a given, either, thanks to the Russian veto on the Security Council.

These seemingly intractable questions filled my head. I barely knew where to start. I decided to set as many hares running as I could, firing off emails and making calls to every UK government and international contact I had. My resolve to help Abu Waseem and his colleagues was renewed every time I heard from one of them via WhatsApp, which was often in the last frenzied weeks of 2016.

NOVEMBER 28, 2016

ALEPPO DOCTOR 1: Hello Dr David, please work quickly to let us go out of Aleppo, we are so worried and afraid.

ME: OK, I will come back to you shortly, how many people do you think will leave if I came for you?

ALEPPO DOCTOR 2: I think all medical staff will go out and most people, I think 100,000, it should be as soon as possible.

ALEPPO DOCTOR 3: Dr David the situation here is so terrible. Civilians moved from districts where regime enter our district . . . People in roads there is not enough houses for them . . . In every hour more and more civilians escaping from regime . . . We think more than 100,000 civilians want to leave besieged Aleppo to north . . . Please doctor if you can press quickly to save us . . . Because in every hour the situation becomes much worse.

The doctors in Aleppo were also getting all sorts of information through social media from many different sources; not all of it was accurate and sometimes they'd hear things before I did. I did my best to reassure them and pass on any snippets that were coming my way about attempts to render the regime corridors more palatable to those stuck inside the besieged city.

NOVEMBER 29

ALEPPO DOCTOR 3: Dr David I want to tell you something so important about corridor: in previous times when Russia asked civilians to move out of besieged Aleppo there was no guarantee that the corridor will be safe (as you know Dr civilians here don't trust regime and Russia) . . . It is so important for civilians to have international guarantee that corridor will be safe. The situation breaking down quickly . . . Regime capturing civilians and send them to a large detained [area] near Aleppo airport. Please help the rest.

ME: Are you OK, there are some movements to make corridor safe for you. Do you think that al-Nusra Front will cause problems for you leaving?

ALEPPO DOCTOR 1: How will leaving . . . arrange with al-Nusra? Who will sponsor evacuation? UN, the British government? Is this safe??

ME: We are meeting today with UK government and UN and I will let you know. Someone said that they thought al-Nusra may stop it, in your opinion is that a possibility? Should I speak to them as well?

ALEPPO DOCTOR 1: No one can stop us . . . Please go on.

On the day I received the texts above, November 29, the regime dropped more leaflets over east Aleppo: "This is the last hope . . . Save yourselves, if you don't leave these areas quickly, YOU WILL BE ANNIHILATED. We have left an open passageway for you to leave. Make a decision . . . Save yourselves. You know that everyone has left you alone to face your doom."

I got in touch with the Foreign & Commonwealth Office (FCO) in London, who in turn were in direct communication with the United Nations. The key man there was Kevin Kennedy, the regional humanitarian coordinator for the crisis in Syria. More general top-level discussions were also taking place independently between John Kerry, the Secretary of State, and Sergey Lavrov, the Russian Foreign Minister—the US and Russia were co-chairs of the International Syria Support Group, an organization of which the

UN, the EU, and other countries were members, and which was pursuing broader talks about how to bring the civil war to an end.

The FCO told me the UN route was completely blocked because of the Russian veto; there was nothing they could do. I was also told that the FCO's hands were tied: they would help with advice and information, but they couldn't get involved. As it turned out, though, my contact at the FCO proved extremely helpful—we began to exchange emails in which I would float some crazy idea or other and he would respond with energy and enthusiasm. I was encouraged at finding someone who seemed to be on my wavelength, at least. He also advised me how to go about approaching the Russians—as a private citizen I couldn't just turn up at the embassy on my own, but had to go through a fairly circuitous route involving the current Dean of the Diplomatic Corps, the longest-serving foreign ambassador to the Court of St. James, who happened to be the Kuwaiti ambassador, Khaled al-Duwaisan.

And so I began to bang on the door of the Russian Embassy, putting forward the case that the bombing had to stop to allow some sort of humanitarian evacuation, and that I was sure the doctors in Aleppo wouldn't leave via the corridors the Russians had put in place.

NOVEMBER 30

ALEPPO DOCTOR 1: Hello Dr David, Russia says that she agreed to open safe [but still regime] corridor to enter aid. Is that true? And does it include evacuation, medical staff or not?

ME: Yes looks as if Russia has agreed. Awaiting regime response. Negotiations happening within Aleppo city council so optimistic, but wait for me to confirm.

ALEPPO DOCTOR 2: Thanks Dr, we will wait and hope that we will have this guarantee . . . In fact in the last two days most injuries we treated were civilians when they were trying to move to regime . . . Even the corridor is unsafe but civilians forced due

> to bombs and hunger to try this corridor (in fact they are escaping from death to death) an example is what you saw yesterday: pictures of victims dead on road with their bags.

But on December 1, I was sent an email from the head of the Russian foreign policy team in London. It quoted at length from a briefing note by Lieutenant-General Sergei Rudskoy, chief of Russian military operations. He claimed, among other things, that more than 90,000 civilians had already been "freed" from Aleppo; that the wounded were receiving medical help; that all remaining males over the age of twelve had been "mobilized by insurgents"—that is, were working actively against the regime. Most incredibly of all, I was informed that "roads, infrastructure, and social-sphere buildings destroyed by the war are being restored. Electricity and water are being provided. All this creates the conditions for a peaceful life."

I simply did not recognize this parallel universe, which bore no resemblance whatsoever to the picture I was getting from my colleagues in Aleppo.

DECEMBER 1

ALEPPO DOCTOR 1: What do you think Dr . . . is evacuation of medical staff possible?

ME: Yes, but wait a bit.

ALEPPO DOCTOR 1: OK. We are so worried and afraid.

DECEMBER 2

ME: How are you today my dear friend? Lots of behind-the-scenes negotiations.

ALEPPO DOCTOR 1: We are fine, thank you. How are negotiations going? What do you think?

ME: So glad to hear that, so glad. Negotiations with UN, I am banging on everybody's door. Slowly things are happening. Keep safe and far away from the regime corridor.

ALEPPO DOCTOR 3: Thanks a lot Dr David . . . You create hope in my soul again. I was very sad today almost want to cry thinking about my wife and my little daughter: I did not see them four months ago . . . Death around us makes my heart very weak . . . Nurse wake me today early to see patient seventy years old cluster fragment injury enters upper lip and out from his neck causing a very severe injury. He was trembling in the emergency room because of cold . . . You know Dr I am thirty-two years old . . . I didn't see Syrian civilians in this situation ever before . . . War is a crime, civilians all hate it . . .

From all reports, it appeared that there were around five hundred children who needed to be evacuated. This was definitely the hook for any negotiation, and the focus of my efforts apart from Abu Waseem and his colleagues. The problem was, where were they going to go? And, of course, members of their family would have to go with them. From talking to my doctors it was obvious they were very nervous about going anywhere associated with the regime. They had to leave by a route that would be agreeable to all parties. But which one? Negotiations with the ICRC, the Syrian Red Crescent, and the United Nations continued.

DECEMBER 3

ME: Working on trying to get doctors out to Bab al-Hawa. Can you let me know what is happening, where you are, I need information.

ALEPPO DOCTOR 1: Huge clashes in the front. We are in Kallasa neighborhood. So so worried.

ME: Are you all there?

ALEPPO DOCTOR 2: Yes all doctors from M1, M2 and M10.

ALEPPO DOCTOR 3: The general situation is bad, regime allies put all their efforts trying to advance in the rest of east Aleppo . . . The shelling is very heavy . . . After two days of no-fly because of bad weather today planes returned to bombing the city and as you see in media all living needs in besieged Aleppo are very difficult to reach. The medical situation becomes more complex. We run out of most of the important medical elements, today we start doing operation without oxygen, day after day our medical service becomes worse and in a very quick manner. For me, I am now in a small basement, we convert it to a very small hospital, trying to save as much as we can of civilians . . . The operation room where I do surgeries is just 3 m x 3 m . . . We are trying to keep this tiny hospital secret in order not to be targeted.

ABU WASEEM: There are too many injuries every day, too many abdominal and vascular injuries. Today there were five vascular at the same time and here just Abu Hozaifa to help them. One day we did seventy surgical procedures.

I kept up the pressure and found myself being copied in on various high-level emails, but it soon became obvious that nothing could break the deadlock between the UN and Russia. Meanwhile, the enclave in Aleppo got steadily smaller, with no letups in the bombing.

DECEMBER 4

ALEPPO DOCTOR 3: Huge amounts of airstrikes targeted Aleppo today . . . This picture of a child is an example of many injuries received today. Doctor, the regime allies every day advancing on ground over victims' bodies . . . Today the Internet cut off for six hours and I am now online through the final Internet route . . . The next few days will be difficult . . . I don't know if I will die, be arrested or go out from this hell . . . Dr David I want to send you my personal ID, maybe will benefit if the regime arrest me. I don't think I can escape without [being captured] . . . Because as a doctor the regime look for me as a terrorist. By the way in all my life I didn't hold a gun and almost all victims we treat are civilians. I am broken inside. Dr David can I send your phone number to my wife . . . She will contact you in case of emergency.

There were some media reports coming out of Aleppo, especially on Channel 4 News, who had gotten ahold of video footage of the horror inside the hospitals and outside on the streets. It was devastating. I continued to lobby TV and radio stations, arguing that the regime's offensive was in breach of international humanitarian law.

DECEMBER 5

ME: Please don't give up. We are still working hard, there are other routes and we are trying them. How is the situation at the moment? I am going on the TV.

ALEPPO DOCTOR 1: Shelling all the time, we managed just a little of casualties. No blood units. No fresh plasma. No oxygen generator. It's horrible situation. We need safe corridor to evacuate civilians. Please help us.

ME: I understand. Am trying to get you a UN safe corridor. Keep safe.

ALEPPO DOCTOR 3: As always planes in sky . . . Bombs everywhere . . . Emergency room full . . . So horrible when victims

> dead on roads and there is no one [to remove them] leaving dead bodies for cats and dogs. Most of the ambulances are out of service due to heavy bombing . . . One of the nurses who works in the last ICU here in besieged Aleppo tells me that in the last three days his full crowded ICU only one patient survive, the rest dead.

Around this time, the plates began to shift. I cannot divulge the specifics, but doors began to open. It was suggested that it might be possible for me to get direct access to President Putin in Moscow, to press the case for a ceasefire on humanitarian grounds. I went back to the Russian Embassy and asked them to arrange for me to fly to Moscow and discuss the situation directly with him. I couldn't believe that he would carry on with the bombing if he was faced with the evidence of what was happening in Aleppo, naive as that sounds. But I was told that the situation was changing too rapidly—a Russian field hospital in west Aleppo had just been shelled by the rebels, and two Russian doctors had died. There were humanitarian catastrophes on both sides, they argued—as if that somehow undermined my case.

And then there was another, even more unexpected, development. It was a Tuesday afternoon and I was in the middle of an operation. My cell phone rang and a nurse held up the phone to my ear. A well-educated English voice asked me to meet him at a coffee shop in central London—he had some helpful information for me.

As soon as I had finished my list, I cycled off to meet my contact, who told me, unbelievably, that it might be possible for me to make my case directly to President Assad in Damascus. He gave me various telephone numbers and I was told that if I called at a particular time early the following morning, Assad would listen to what I had to say.

"This is the time when you need to call," my contact said. "You should say that you are a surgical colleague from London who works at Imperial College. You knew him when he was at the Western Eye Hospital in 1993. That will give you an in to speak to him."

While I prepared for this potentially significant shift in the negotiations, I checked in with my doctors again.

DECEMBER 6

ME: How are things today my friend?

ALEPPO DOCTOR 1: Too bad . . . Massacres and no medication . . . Regime is advancing.

ME: Do you want to talk to Channel 4 News by Skype? But I don't want to put you into a difficult position.

ALEPPO DOCTOR 1: I can't talk to media . . . Excuse me.

ME: I understand, no problem.

ALEPPO DOCTOR 1: What you think Dr David . . . Is evacuation possible?

ME: I'm going to talk to someone who may be able to stop the bombing and help with the evacuation. The meeting [the Assad call] is on for tomorrow morning.

ALEPPO DOCTOR 1: I pray all the time. Rebels decided to leave Aleppo city. I hope that this news help us to get out of the city.

ME: That is good news. We are in discussions [with the UN] to send a convoy to pick up injured children and those doctors that care for them (and that will be you and your colleagues) hopefully as early as Friday if my plan works.

At six o'clock on the morning of Wednesday, December 7, I made my first telephone call directly to President Assad's office. It was about an hour before I was put through. Finally a gruff, military-sounding voice said curtly in Arabic, "What?"

I had a fluent Arabic speaker with me and, through him, I explained who I was—carefully omitting the fact that I'd been working in east Aleppo—and said I wanted to speak to President Assad to discuss the evacuation of injured children from Aleppo.

"Who are you?" the gruff voice said, quite aggressively. "UN?"

I explained that I was part of an international humanitarian effort to secure a ceasefire. I then said I'd like to speak in English, and the voice said, "OK, speak. We're all here." I asked if Assad was there and was told he was, but that under no circumstances would the president speak to me in person—he would only listen on speakerphone.

I took a deep breath and launched in. I had no idea if Assad genuinely was listening or whether he was even in the room at the other end of the line, but I knew I had to try. I put the case purely on humanitarian grounds, playing on the fact that he too had trained as a doctor, and was signed up to the Hippocratic oath that all physicians abide by. I told him that there were around five hundred children who needed immediate evacuation from east Aleppo. I asked him directly to call a ceasefire so that they could be moved—the UN had told me they would make vehicles available to escort them out. The gruff voice came back on, skeptical, noncommittal; they would not agree to the use of UN vehicles.

I repeated the arguments, and was amazed when a different voice came on the line, this time in English, much more softly spoken and cultured. He said, "OK, welcome, goodbye," and the call ended. Was this Assad himself? I will never know. Nor did I know what, if anything, had been achieved, but it felt like progress. I was told to call again the following day.

DECEMBER 7

ME: Hopefully ceasefire very soon.

ALEPPO DOCTOR 1: Please, Doctor . . . Do everything to save us.

ME: Try to keep safe. There is a lot of work going on behind the scenes. Hopefully the next day or so there will be a corridor open

> to the north. I will see you very shortly. Keep safe my friend. Be in touch if you have Internet.
>
> ALEPPO DOCTOR 2: We are so worried, regime is advancing.
>
> ALEPPO DOCTOR 3: Regime become very close to us . . . We will close our field hospital and flee to the final district where the rebels are. I maybe cannot be in touch with you Dr David.

With the regime advancing on all sides, the area of Aleppo not yet controlled by them was shrinking by the day. Soon it was a matter of one or two square miles. Unexpectedly, the UN received an email from the Aleppo Leadership Council, which comprised the various rebel groups now known as the "Armed Operating Groups" (AOGs), asking for a five-day ceasefire. It was a plea from the inside—the bombing had become too intense. The email caused a great stir and allowed Secretary of State Kerry to push again for the ceasefire with his Russian counterpart.

I was copied into an email from the UN's Kevin Kennedy, which said that the Armed Operating Groups might be able to hold out for a maximum of five more days, but that some were expecting the city to fall as soon as the following day. There were reports that Assad's elite unit, the 4th Division, was leading the offensive; there were rumors of revenge killings by the Iranian militias tasked with taking over the "liberated" areas. Some estimates put the number of civilians still trapped in the besieged enclave at 100,000; the percentage of these who needed medical care was not clear.

Kevin warned that the window of opportunity was fast closing. He made the case for the continuation of the Kerry-Lavrov talks and also raised the concern about how doctors, medical staff, and NGOs would be treated—would they be allowed to leave, or stay and continue their work in safety? He concluded:

> David, if you get through to Assad, this is an issue that you should raise; he should make a public statement to the effect that

> people are secure and are free to go about their way. Lastly, if there is no joy tomorrow on the call to Assad, consider making a public statement as to the elaborate arrangements that have been put in place, ready to go, to treat critically injured children. The UN has made dozens of statements without much effect. A public statement from private operators puts the ball in their court and might just force them to react.

I suddenly felt under a lot of pressure. The telephone calls to President Assad's office seemed ever more urgent. I called every morning. I would get up at six, call the numbers I'd been given, and wait to be put through. If I wasn't put through, I'd call back until I was. Sometimes I'd get through and General Gruff would say "What?" before letting me speak for a bit and then hanging up. Then, during one call, when I said, for what must have been the hundredth time, that the UN had a convoy of buses waiting and that they had to confirm a ceasefire, there was a shift.

"No UN buses," I was told. "Our buses only."

Did this mean they had agreed? It was impossible to tell. All I could do was to keep pushing, keep calling.

DECEMBER 8

ME: Are you ready to go? How many doctors are ready to go, how many children do you think are ready to go? Can you give me this information as soon as possible.

ALEPPO DOCTOR 1: Most doctors want to leave, thirty to forty. We are in Kallasa and Sukkari. Regime is advancing. I think 400–500 children should go out.

ME: OK you'll be hearing very shortly from the WHO [World Health Organization] who is in west Aleppo. They will tell you what to do. Call these numbers. Tell them that I told you to speak to them, they will coordinate with you.

ALEPPO DOCTOR 1: OK.

ME: Trying to get you safe passage to the north today.

ALEPPO DOCTOR 1: Oh God . . . Save us and get us out to our family.

ME: I want to know whether you feel able to leave where you are at moment. Is it north via Castello Road or is there another road that you think is better?

ALEPPO DOCTOR 1: Castello Road.

ME: OK, do you think it's best to pick you up where you are? Would you want to be picked up where you are?

ALEPPO DOCTOR 1: Is not a problem . . . In Kallasa or Sukkari.

ME: Has the bombing stopped?

ALEPPO DOCTOR 3: In the last hour, tens of injuries in the emergency room and bombs don't stop. He hit us with chlorine, what is happening, oh my God, chlorine children crying coughing and my God my God. Regime wants to kill us all.

Behind the scenes, the high-level email discussions continued. These exchanges led to an offer from another contact to get a message directly to President Putin. Could he arrange for a ceasefire to allow the five hundred children trapped in east Aleppo to leave? I made the case, as I was doing to Assad's office, that it was about presenting a picture to the world of themselves as humanitarians rather than warmongers. To my amazement, I was told that Putin agreed to suspend hostilities, but it wasn't clear when, or for how long.

DECEMBER 9

ALEPPO DOCTOR 1: Dr David we are ready . . . Please tell them to help to stop bombing and get us out.

ME: Do you think that the children can be sent via designated corridors to the west and the medical staff and sick patients moved to the north?

ALEPPO DOCTOR 1: We can't send anyone to the regime.

In west Aleppo the heads of the ICRC, Syrian Red Crescent, and the World Health Organization were negotiating with the Russian commanders on the ground to discuss various crossing points through which civilians and the injured might be able to leave. Of course, the Russians and the Syrian regime manned all these crossings. Safe passage for both civilians and doctors from rebel-held areas through territory now controlled by the regime was still a huge issue. They needed assurances that they wouldn't be arrested on their way to the neutral zone we were trying to set up, where they could be picked up by various NGOs and taken to the north. But again there were positive signs—during the meeting one of the Russian generals had taken a telephone call confirming that there would soon be a ceasefire.

DECEMBER 10

ME: How are you doing today? Let me know what the situation is like today my dear friend. I need to pass the info to the UN.

ALEPPO DOCTOR 1: Massive shelling . . . Today is bunker busting bombs.

ME: OK, we are trying and trying.

ALEPPO DOCTOR 3: The helicopter dropped chlorine container directly over a building . . . It was very panic moment . . . Thank God we still are alive . . . Today aircraft and helicopter activities very high and we feel five to six times ground shake because of bunker rockets (maybe Russian aircraft) . . . for patients evacuation, nothing happened, Russia want patients to walk 1 km to regime region where ambulances wait for them! Dr David give me your views . . . What will happen to us, I feel every day I am closer to death.

The delicacy of the situation wasn't helped when the Armed Operating Groups launched a mortar attack on western Aleppo, killing dozens of people and injuring three hundred. This was not good.

I began relaying all the WhatsApp messages I was receiving to Kevin Kennedy, who then forwarded them on to the State Department in Washington so everybody could read what it was really like on the inside.

DECEMBER 11

ALEPPO DOCTOR 1: We have a list of patients and sent it to UN.

ME: I have said all the calls must go through me, so wait to hear from me.

ALEPPO DOCTOR 1: It must be arranged with rebels Dr David.

ME: There are negotiations with somebody call Farouk [in charge of the Armed Operating Groups] – do you know him?

ALEPPO DOCTOR 1: Yes yes . . . That's good.

ME: Is it worth me talking to him as well?

ALEPPO DOCTOR 1: If negotiations between UN and Farouk, it is OK and no need to talk to him.

ME: I am sorry but the Russian/US talks in Geneva failed again. I'm working very hard to get a ceasefire for you working with lots of politicians. If we can get a ceasefire then the UN will take you.

ALEPPO DOCTOR 1: Go ahead . . . Bless you. Do you know why talks failed? Rebels are agree to leave . . . I am afraid that US does bad situation to disable any agreement to annihilate us . . . What do you think?

ME: I don't know. I am so frustrated. But still trying. Trying at this moment to get [another] message to Putin, but when they agreed to a small ceasefire last week, regime didn't stop bombing. But we are trying again. Need to get Putin to tell Assad stop bombing. When I know the time for ceasefire then that will be the time to move. OK?

ALEPPO DOCTOR 3: The situation is like doomsday . . . A very aggressive war against civilians . . . Even chlorine every day helicopters dropped chlorine containers . . . What happened to humanity when women children and elders walk on foot between bombs, some died on the road and left alone for animals to eat them . . . Some reach regime region where allies are ready to arrest men and put them again on the front lines . . . Yesterday, Russian aircraft hit Alhajj Bridge with bunker bombs in order to cut it . . . Besieged Aleppo sky are always full with helicopters and aircraft . . . Yesterday the helicopter didn't drop bombs because there was a Russian aircraft . . . Patient stories are same, two days ago we received a ten-year-old girl from under the rubble and is always a girl alone with no father nor mother . . . Try to give her treatment as I can and start to take care of her, hoping someone will come and ask about her name . . . In the evening, regime hit our medical point with chlorine and [so we] remove patients to second medical point . . . Imagine Dr when

> she went to the other medical point a nurse asked a woman to give the girl a place beside her in the bed, and suddenly the woman shouted My daughter my daughter . . .

I became desperate again, realizing that we really were running out of time and that every avenue was being blocked. Surely somebody should be able to do something to stop this? The situation was getting even worse, with chlorine bombs forcing people out of their cellars, as chlorine is heavier than air. And then when they did emerge from their underground shelters, they were targeted with shells and rocket fire. Every news outlet ran pictures of the devastation and the human suffering. It was horrific.

On December 12, I received a telephone call from the Russian Embassy asking me to contact them urgently. I spoke to my senior consulate adviser, who said they had been contacted by Moscow—there would definitely be a ceasefire, I was told, and President Putin had given his assurances that this would happen. I was told not to go public with this news just yet.

Andrew Mitchell had put in for a second emergency debate and again I was in the chamber of the House of Commons to hear it. Just before the debate began I received a live WhatsApp video from inside Aleppo. It was Abu Waseem, looking like a homeless person, wearing several layers of clothes on his head and body. The temperature was minus ten, they had no food left, no water, and only one generator. He asked me how I was. I was close to tears, but tried to stay strong for him.

"We will get you out," I said. "Just wait."

"Thank you, my friend," was his reply, but I knew it was probably the last time I would ever see him if the promised ceasefire fell through.

After the debate, having thanked Andrew Mitchell for all he had done, I got on my bicycle to go back to work. Amid a mass of traffic near Victoria, I felt my phone vibrate in my pocket. Something made me stop and fish it out, with cold drizzle blurring the screen.

I let out a yelp—it was a message from Kevin Kennedy saying that a ceasefire had come into force from all sides. It had been confirmed a short time after the emergency debate had finished. The regime was supplying a convoy of green buses, and these would ferry people out. Another email came from Kevin shortly after: "David, your advocacy has brought the issue to international attention . . . let's just hope it brings positive results." He later informed me that a deal had been reached between the Turkish and Russian presidents to allow all civilians and rebel fighters to leave Aleppo.

I could not quite believe it, but it seemed to be happening. My friends were finally going to be safe.

DECEMBER 15

ALEPPO DOCTOR 1: I have left Aleppo and I am with my family . . . I thank you so much for everything you did.

ALEPPO DOCTOR 3: Hello Dr David . . . I just arrived home at 3 a.m. . . . It was so special moment when I saw my family for the first time in many months.

ABU WASEEM: Thank you, we are so sad we will leave Aleppo for ever.

ME: I know my friend but you are alive, I am so happy.

ABU WASEEM: Hello my friend we are now out of Aleppo, thank you very much.

Long lines of green regime buses had arrived with ambulances for the sick and injured to take them to the crossing point, where they would be handed over to various NGOs including Syria Relief. The ambulances would take the sick and wounded to hospitals in Idlib.

The next day, Mounir Hakimi called me. The exodus of buses was constant, and there were many wounded people suffering from terrible injuries, as well as frostbite and psychological trauma from the constant bombing. Would I join him in Syria? Of course, I jumped at the opportunity.

I was in Tel Aviv when I got the call. Elly and I had flown there prior to running a HEST course in Gaza with the International Committee of the

Red Cross, with support from our foundation. We immediately canceled the course and I left our hotel room at some unearthly hour in the morning to fly to Istanbul, then on to Hatay. There I met Mounir, and we crossed into Syria.

That afternoon Mounir went down to the crossing point at Al-Rashdeen, while I stayed in Bab al-Hawa examining patients who had just been transferred from Aleppo. Mounir later told me how extraordinary it had been to stand at the crossing and watch people coming out of Aleppo on the green regime buses. As they crossed from the horror of their besieged and devastated city to freedom, he was struck by how surreal it was to see Russian soldiers help them down from the buses, when only hours earlier they had been shooting at them.

That evening, Mounir suggested that we drive to a local restaurant, rather than eating at the hospital as we usually did. It was snowing heavily, and the journey took about half an hour. Because the security situation was still so febrile, when we got to the restaurant I was smuggled in through the back door wearing a large woolen hat as a disguise. We went into a large dining room that seemed to be screened off from the rest of the restaurant. Suddenly, a curtain lifted and there they all were—around thirty of the doctors who had got out of Aleppo, including Abu Waseem and Abu Hozaifa. It was one of the most emotional reunions of my life, and a wonderfully happy end to a hellish period for them. So many people had worked for weeks on end to make this happen—the British government, the UN, dignitaries, and go-betweens, and—of course—the people in the shadows. I was so grateful to all of them, and so thrilled that our persistence had paid off.

Abu Waseem stayed with me for a week, which we spent operating on many of his patients who needed refinements to their amputations or reconstructive surgery. It was fantastic to have my student by my side again.

One little girl in particular touched my heart. Her name was Maram and she was just five months old. Her mother and father had been killed going through one of the crossing points to west Aleppo. She had terrible injuries from fragmentation wounds to her leg, hand, and arm, and was obviously in a great deal of pain. She was very septic and could easily have died without proper wound management, and she also needed urgent realignment of her fractured bones. It was our last day; Mounir tended to her orthopedic injuries and I dealt with all her soft-tissue wounds. I worried that her injuries were too serious for her to survive, but we did as much as we could.

The following day was Christmas Eve. I went to find Maram just before I crossed the border back to Turkey, on my way home. I scoured the wards but she was not there. Some of the doctors and nurses I spoke to knew nothing about her, so I assumed the worst: she must have died in the night and simply been taken away, another victim of this senseless war.

When I got back to London, I drove straight down to Devon to meet my family, finally arriving at three in the morning. I counted my blessings that Christmas Day as I held Molly and Elly close. How very lucky we are.

It is hard to be optimistic about Syria. My colleagues and others like them will carry on their work, because they are courageous and dedicated. But it is difficult to see a positive outcome for the country unless major political pressure is brought to bear. As we have seen in more recent months, in eastern Ghouta and elsewhere, the imperative to get Assad's regime to behave more moderately is as strong as ever. My heart bleeds for Syria's people and I hope and pray that a way toward peace will soon be found.

As ever, it is the tiny beacons of light amid the darkness that give us hope. A couple of months after my return from Bab al-Hawa, the BBC contacted me. Unbelievably, they had found Maram in Turkey. Would I like to visit her?

I flew via Istanbul to Hatay, and then drove to Reyhanlı. A BBC camera crew came with me and captured the extraordinary moment when I saw that brave little girl smiling up at me, alive and well. "Well, well, well," were the words I said when I looked at her. "I've brought you a dolly." The look on that little girl's face radiating hope, happiness, pure innocence, love, and possible forgiveness epitomized all that is good about this world. As the Koran says in Surah 5:32: *Whoever saves a life, it shall be as though he had saved the lives of all mankind.*

She, and all the other children and innocent victims of conflict the world over, is the reason I do what I do.

AFTERWORD
BY ELEANOR NOTT

Heroism is a consistent theme in the stories human beings tell one another: people of great strength doing remarkable things.

Second only to stories of romantic love, the tale of the hero undertaking a mission, overcoming adversity, and emerging triumphant has adorned cave walls and filled library shelves for centuries. Heroic stories give us hope, make us feel better about our sometimes-wretched world, and serve as inspiration and aspiration. We may not have those qualities ourselves, but knowing they are out there gives us comfort.

Society demands heroes, but we don't necessarily want them to be too human. We don't want messiness. To remain pleasing to us they should exist in a sphere of goodness and virtue we ourselves find impossible to attain. At the first hint of failing, the first chink in the armor, the bubble is burst and the search for perfection begins afresh.

Love, like surgery, isn't always tidy, and it isn't always easy. In many ways rushing in and out of war zones is easier than the day-in, day-out normality of home life. You won't always be the hero and savior—there will be routine, boredom, and difficult conversations.

I often have to remind myself what an adjustment married life and fatherhood must be for David, someone who has lived so much of his life on the razor's edge and in a fair degree of emotional isolation.

Our beginning was sometimes painful, as he has described in these pages. Knowing what I do about him, though, I at least had some insight into why he acted as he did. I am grateful to him for showing true bravery and telling me things about his life that he had not shared with anyone before. They helped me to understand.

To see the best of David is to observe him with two very different groups of people. The first are the Syrian doctors he loves like brothers, and the second are his daughters.

. . .

Throughout 2016, as the situation in Aleppo spiraled ever downward, David was consumed by an all-encompassing desire to end the devastation being wrought on the doctors and civilians of that city. His phone burned with images of what Russian and Syrian bombs and bullets were doing to soft little bodies. There were dark nights of the soul, hours spent hunched over a laptop and tapping into a cell phone. It was difficult to engage him on any subject other than Syria.

When, after months of advocacy, the buses started rolling out of Aleppo and into Idlib, I told him to go with my blessing to his friends. The camaraderie he has, not only with the doctors he trained in Aleppo but with the Syrian expatriate community in the UK, is a thing of beauty. I can only imagine how moved he must have been to see them all again that December. It was so cold they gave him a heavy brown sheepskin coat. If he's working late at home now, he'll sometimes crash on our sofa downstairs and I'll come down to find him fast asleep under the Syrian coat, with its small burn mark down the back from where he got too close to a gas fire. I wonder what he's dreaming about; I hope it's a dream of eating ice cream at the last gelateria in Aleppo with his friends, or driving fast between hospitals with Abu Abdul's Kalashnikov on the dashboard to deter anyone who might want to stop them.

It's not too much to say he loves them. In his association with the doctors of free Aleppo he found companionship, a sense of purpose, meaning, and mission and was moved by their kindness to him. We all want to make a contribution, to feel that our lives have meaning. In the absence of any family at that time, the doctors gave him just that.

It amuses and delights David that Abu Waseem calls him "Abu Molly," meaning, of course, "Father of Molly" in Arabic. One of my greatest joys is seeing David contend with the two tiny people who assail him as he arrives through our front door. We listen out for Daddy's motorcycle, or the screech of his bicycle's brakes, then the door is flung open and Molly and Elizabeth will scramble to take their places in his arms. He is a warm, gentle, and devoted father. I sometimes listen through the door as he reads Molly her bedtime story; and when Elizabeth was ill he stayed up with her through the night, holding her in his arms because it made her feel safe and secure, even though it meant he had no sleep himself.

Early on it became clear that David's humanitarian work is an intrinsic part of who he is. Although I found this hard at first, having worried so desperately when he was working in Syria, I fully support him in what he does—to do otherwise would not only deny David his passion but also deprive the world of his skills, which are so desperately needed.

From the moment we met I started to turn over in my mind how we could train more doctors in the surgical skills they need to save lives in the most war-torn and poorest places on earth. I set up the David Nott Foundation so we could raise funds to support doctors to come to the UK and be trained by David on the course he directs at the Royal College of Surgeons of England: Surgical Training for Austere Environments. If we raised enough, we could also run courses abroad, take our training right to the front line where it is needed most.

While pregnant with Molly, I set up camp at our kitchen table with my laptop and a stack of Charity Commission documents. I wrote us a constitution, recruited some trustees, and set up a bank account. On David's birthday in 2015, I received notification that we had been granted charitable status. Two weeks later, Molly was born.

The David Nott Foundation has grown extraordinarily since our early beginnings. As we are a young charity, every donation feels personal, an expression of faith in us, and we take that responsibility very seriously.

In the last four years our Foundation teams have trained more than 750 doctors during thirteen Hostile Environment Surgical Training (HEST) courses overseas. We have held four courses for Syrian doctors since 2016, in Gaziantep, Turkey, and in Idlib, Syria. We have also been to Yemen, twice, at the invitation of Médecins Sans Frontières, and to Gaza with the Red Cross. We have taught further courses in the Palestinian Territories, Iraq, Libya, Lebanon, Cameroon, and Kenya. We have also undertaken surgical missions to Lebanon and Cox's Bazar, Bangladesh, to treat Rohingya refugees fleeing the violence in Myanmar.

We have welcomed sixty-two scholars to London to attend the Surgical Training for Austere Environments (STAE) course. We award scholarships to attend this prestigious course to doctors who show great promise in the field of humanitarian surgery, and we pay for their course fee, flights, visas, and accommodations. There is now a virtuous circle whereby when we teach a HEST course abroad we get a flurry of scholarship applications and similarly our scholars invite us to their home cities to teach.

Our first substantial grant was from the Open Society Foundations for a state-of-the-art simulator mannequin. This invaluable teaching aid replicates exactly the anatomy of a human and allows the faculty to demonstrate operations and procedures. We have entered into a partnership with one of the world's leading telecommunications groups' charitable arm to produce an app that will be a resource for doctors anywhere in the world. It will comprise a library of David's surgical videos and expertise, demonstrations, and a community function enabling doctors to ask for advice and share experiences.

Surgery hasn't had the profile of other health issues such as communicable or preventable diseases. Yet surgically treatable conditions kill 17 million people each year; more than tuberculosis, malaria, and HIV/AIDS combined, according to a study in *The Lancet*. We therefore seek to promote the skillful and safe practice of surgery in low-resource or war-torn settings as well as advocate for the rights of the medical victims of conflict and the doctors who strive to care for them.

There is no shortage of need for the training we provide. In the coming years we want to expand our reach and deepen our links with the communities we have been privileged to help. We want to build regional hubs and be recognized as the authority in teaching surgical skills for austere environments, raising the standard of humanitarian surgery worldwide.

David embodies the truly heroic, if we will but allow our heroes the vulnerability and humanity that make them real people. A wise priest at the Catholic church where I was baptized and confirmed once said, "Go for the best and be prepared to work for it." It has always stuck with me. I wouldn't want our daughters to miss real love in search of a romantic mirage; I am glad I didn't either.

A hero all the more worthy of love *because* of his vulnerabilities. My extraordinary, complicated, beloved David.

ACKNOWLEDGMENTS

When I returned from a six-week surgical mission to Aleppo in 2014 I gave an interview to Eddie Mair on the BBC Radio 4 *PM* program. It was a time when the world seemed to have forgotten about the Syrian civil war. It rarely made the news and I was determined to make people listen, having seen the most horrific injuries day in, day out during my time in Aleppo.

After the interview's airdate, which took place almost a year to the day after a previous one I had given to Eddie Mair, I started to get some emails from various literary agents asking if I had ever considered writing a book. The truth was, I had not. I have authored several medical textbooks but hadn't ever contemplated writing more broadly, or personally, about my experiences as a doctor in the UK and abroad. Maybe, I thought, this would be an effective way to tell the world what was happening in Syria.

It was a cold, gray afternoon in January 2015 when Andrew Gordon came to see me in my office. Elly, whom I was to marry two weeks later, was there as ever, providing the usual brightness, good humor, and energy she does to everything. We liked Andrew instantly and he has been my constant guide through the process of writing the book; unfailingly kind, supportive, and constructive. He took the "word salad" I handed him in January 2018 and tamed it to make it something I am very proud of. I cannot thank him enough.

In addition to Andrew, Nicky Lund has handled my story with sensitivity and thoughtfulness and we are grateful to all the team at David Higham Associates.

From our first meeting with Macmillan/Picador we were impressed by the dynamism of Georgina Morley and her team. I knew that with them the book would be in safe hands and they have been a pleasure to work with, making the book better at every step.

I have quietly pursued my humanitarian missions abroad since 1993 when I first went to Sarajevo with Médecins Sans Frontières. The admiration

I have for those who take time out from their lives of comfort and security to use their skills to help others abroad is enormous. The staff and volunteers for MSF, the International Committee of the Red Cross, and Syria Relief deserve the utmost respect, and I have made lasting friendships from my work with these remarkable people: Harald Veen, Haydar Alwash, Rachel Craven, Pete Mathew, Carlos Pilasi Menichetti, and countless others.

I am indebted to my colleagues and employers at the London hospitals where I work for always allowing me to dash off to a different part of the world at short notice. At Chelsea and Westminster: Jeremy Booth, Peter Dawson, Daryl Dob, Simon Eccles, Roger Gibson, Rick Keays, James McCall, Zoe Penn, Warwick Radford, Richard Smith, Lesley Watts, and Ron Zeegen. Mark Johnson could not have been kinder to Elly and me throughout both her pregnancies and we will forever be grateful to him and Mark Cox for safely delivering our daughters. At St. Mary's: Chris Aylwin, Nicola Batrick, Mansoor Khan, Usman Jaffer, Nigel Standfield, Mark Wilson, and my vascular surgical colleagues. At the Royal Marsden: Andy Hayes and Dirk Strauss, and at the Lister Hospital: Suzy Jones. Special thanks to my wonderful, long-suffering secretary, Lisa Gray, who masterfully juggles my clinics and lists when I am called away on humanitarian missions. I am very grateful. At Imperial College: Roger Kneebone and Justin Cobb. In the NHS, all the registrars past and present whom I have taught and all the wonderful nurses I have had the pleasure of working with both in the operating rooms and on the wards.

I also have my patients to thank for being, for the most part, incredibly patient with me. I have sometimes had to cancel clinics and lists when a humanitarian emergency required me to travel abroad at short notice. My patients have been not only supportive but incredibly generous in supporting the foundation, which I am very touched by.

I am grateful to the Royal College of Surgeons of England for seeing the worth in the Surgical Training for Austere Environments (STAE) course I direct and for supporting me in delivering it. My friends at the college and in setting up STAE have included: Tony Redmond, Jonathan Barden, Vishy Mahadevan, Martyn Coomber, Francine Alexander, Christine Melidou, Clare Marx, Derek Alderson, and Bernie Ribeiro.

ACKNOWLEDGMENTS

My life started to change when I traveled to Syria that first time. On the further missions I undertook to Aleppo, I met doctors who would become not just friends but something akin to family. They gave me a sense of purpose and I will be forever grateful for the time I spent with them. Abu Waseem, Abu Khalifa, Abu Abdul, Abdulaziz, Abu Mohammadain, Mounir Hakimi, Ghanem Tayara, Ayman Jundi, Louay El-Abed, and Saladin Sawan. I hope I have helped a little, I have always done my best. In Ammar Darwish I found the brother I never had. His quiet, calm, steady presence was my guide through many of the most hazardous moments I have ever experienced. His wonderful wife, Aala El-Khani, instantly took Elly under her wing the moment they met and has been the greatest support to her.

I will always be grateful to Eddie Mair for that first interview I gave to the *PM* program in December 2013. It gave me the time and space to say what was happening in Syria. Listening to that broadcast was the artist Bob and Roberta Smith, one of the most delightful people I have ever met, who took our words and made them into a five-meter-high by four-meter-wide painting that hung in the 2014 Royal Academy Summer Exhibition.

In 2016 I was honored to be asked to do *Desert Island Discs* on BBC Radio 4. I was in the studio for about two hours and deeply uncertain, when the recording finished, about how I would come across when it was broadcast. The response to the program was astonishing and I remain deeply humbled by the kind messages that I still receive from people saying that the words I said and music I chose meant something to them. I am so grateful to Cathy Drysdale, Kirsty Young, and all their team for giving me the opportunity.

Desert Island Discs gave a great boost to the charity I established with Elly, the David Nott Foundation. We established the foundation to train doctors in the surgical skills they need to provide relief and assistance in areas affected by conflict and catastrophe. We provide scholarships for doctors to visit the UK and be trained by me on the course I direct at the Royal College of Surgeons of England, and also take teaching courses abroad. We have trained doctors on the Turkish-Syrian border and in Yemen, Palestine, Iraq, Libya, Lebanon, and Cameroon. I am so grateful to all those who have donated or used their skills to support the foundation; it means the world to me that you see value in what we do. I also owe thanks to trustees past and present and our wonderful patron, Betty Boothroyd.

There have been many people in the media, pressure groups, politics, and the diplomatic community who have sought to raise awareness of the humanitarian situation in Syria. Special thanks must go to the Right Honourable Alistair Burt MP, who has always listened respectfully to my concerns and done his best to help. The Right Honourable Andrew Mitchell MP managed to schedule two emergency debates in the House of Commons to discuss the humanitarian situation in Aleppo. When I first went to see him at his home in 2016, armed as ever with my laptop of photos and evidence of what was happening in the besieged eastern half of the city, he welcomed me in and did everything he could to help. Hamish de Bretton-Gordon and I met through our support for the Syrian doctors and have become great friends. John Sweeney and Saleyha Ahsan have striven to raise the humanitarian situation in Syria in the public consciousness.

Many friends have encouraged me to keep going with writing this book when the scale of my other commitments was slowing me down: Stephen Bowers, Dorothy Byrne, Jamie and Neena Crinnion, Michael and Wendy Feher, Peter Godwin, Phil Goodall, Roger Marwood, Meirion, Alison Moodie, Eleanor and Dorabella Moskovic-Thomas, Andrew Norman, Andy and Jim Rose, Quentin Smith, Neil and Alison Soni, Richard Staughton, and Johnny and Lucy Woods.

In this, as in everything else, my greatest support has been Elly. Along with Molly and Elizabeth, she has been my inspiration. I will always remember dictating sections of the book in summer 2017 with the sleeping infant Elizabeth in my arms, sitting in the roof space of our little house in Hammersmith. Thank-yous also go to my wonderful Welsh aunts, uncles, and cousins, and now also to Elly's equally wonderful family, Steve and Wendy, and June and Jerry.

Going back to the start, I thank the hills, woods, and rivers of Carmarthenshire for their beauty and mysticism, which shaped my childhood and provide my spiritual hinterland and place of peace. I wish that my parents Malcolm and Yvonne were here to share all this with me, and I wish I could thank them for all the love and support they gave me throughout our wonderful years together. They lie together next to my Mamgu and Datcu, high on a hill in a beautiful place called Bryn Moriah, four miles from where it all began.

ABOUT THE FOUNDATION

The David Nott Foundation is a UK-registered charity that delivers the best surgical training to medical professionals operating in austere and hostile environments worldwide, enabling them to save more lives.

We are a humanitarian organization motivated to save the lives of the medical victims of conflict and catastrophe. The most powerful way we believe we can do that is by equipping the doctors who care for them with the skills and knowledge they need to make the right choices for their patients and be better surgeons.

We do this by bringing doctors to the UK to be trained on surgical skills courses and also by taking that teaching to the front line. Using a diverse mix of teaching methods and materials, and led by a world-class faculty of experienced and distinguished surgeons, we strive to make our courses impactful and effective. Our vision is a global network of medical professionals, trained to the highest standards, providing the best care to patients in austere or hostile environments.

To support our work and donate, visit: www.davidnottfoundation.com